T0230567

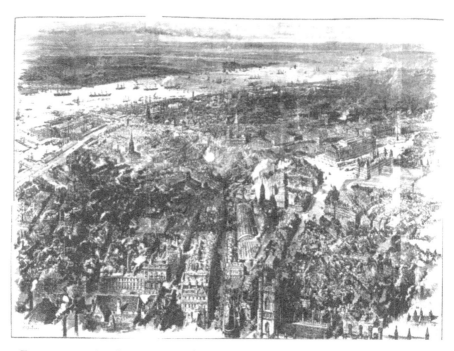

Frontispiece: Bird's eye view of Liverpool by W.L. Wyllie and H.W. Brewer.
Published in the Graphic, 22 August 1885.
By permission of the British Library.

Body and City

Historical Urban Studies

Series Editors: Richard Rodger and Jean-Luc Pinol

Titles in this series include:

Capital Cities and their Hinterlands in Early Modern Europe
edited by Peter Clark and Bernard Lepetit

*Power, Profit and Urban Land: Landownership in Medieval and
Early Modern Northern European Towns*
edited by Finn-Einar Eliassen and Geir Atle Ersland

*Water and European Cities from the Middle ages to the
Nineteenth Century*
edited by Jean-Luc Pinol and Dennis Menjeot

The Built Form of Colonial Cities
Manuel Texeira

Advertising and the European City
edited by Clemens Wischermann and Elliot Shore

*Cathedrals of Urban Modernity:
the First Museums of Contemporary Art, 1800–1930*
J. Pedro Lorente

The Artisan and the European Town, 1500–1900
edited by Geoffrey Crossick

*Urban Fortunes: Property and
Inheritance in the Town, 1700–1900*
edited by Jon Stobart and Alastair Owens

Urban Governance: Britain and Beyond since 1750
edited by R.J. Morris and R.H. Trainor

Body and City

Histories of Urban Public Health

Edited by
Sally Sheard and Helen Power

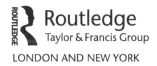

LONDON AND NEW YORK

First published 2000 by Ashgate Publishing

Published 2017 by Routledge
2 Park Square, Milton Park, Abingdon, Oxfordshire OX14 4RN
711 Third Avenue, New York, NY 10017, USA

First issued in paperback 2017

Routledge is an imprint of the Taylor & Francis Group, an informa business

British Library Cataloguing-in-Publication Data
Body and city: histories of urban public health. –
    (Historical urban studies)
    1. Public health – history 2. Urban health – History
    I. Sheard, Sally II. Power, Helen J., 1966–
    362.1'09

US Library of Congress Cataloging-in-Publication Data
The Library of Congress number is: 00-106071

ISBN 13: 978-1-138-27101-2 (pbk)
ISBN 13: 978-1-84014-675-2 (hbk)

Contents

List of figures   vii
List of tables   ix
Notes on contributors   x
Acknowledgements   xiii
General editors' preface   xiv
Preface   xvi

1   Body and city: medical and urban histories of public health   1
    Sally Sheard and Helen Power

2   Ritual and public health in the early medieval city   17
    Peregrine Horden

3   Languages of plague in early modern France   41
    Colin Jones

4   Copenhagen 1711: Danish authorities facing the plague   50
    Peter Christensen

5   Fighting for public health: Dr Duncan and his adversaries,
    1847–63   59
    Paul Laxton

6   Town Hall and Whitehall: sanitary intelligence in Liverpool,
    1840–63   89
    Gerry Kearns

7   Working-class experiences, cholera and public health
    reform in nineteenth-century Switzerland   109
    Flurin Condrau and Jakob Tanner

8   Public health discourses in Birmingham and Gothenburg,
    1890–1920   123
    Marjaana Niemi

9   Choices for town councillors in nineteenth-century Britain:
     investment in public health and its impact on mortality   143
     Robert Millward and Frances Bell

10   Economics and infant mortality decline in German towns,
     1889–1912: household behaviour and public intervention   166
     John Brown

11   The decline of the urban penalty: milk supply and infant
     welfare centres in Germany, 1890s–1920s   194
     Jörg Peter Vögele, Wolfgang Woelk and Silke Fehlemann

Index   215

List of figures

Bird's eye view of Liverpool, 1885   *Frontispiece*

3.1   Three scripts for plague   44

5.1   Liverpool Workhouse and the fever sheds, 1848   73
5.2   Cecil Wray's model lodging houses, 1848   82

6.1   The relations between central and local government in the field of sanitary reform   93
6.2   Sanitary intelligence and the politics of central–local relations   95

8.1   Crude death rates in Birmingham and Gothenburg, 1890–1920   126
8.2   Death rates from pulmonary tuberculosis in Birmingham,1912   130
8.3   Deaths from tuberculosis in Gothenburg, 1904   132

9.1   Capital expenditure out of loans for sanitation and water supply in 36 towns in England and Wales, 1884–1913   151

10.1   Infant mortality in German cities, 1888–1912   167
10.2   The progress of sanitary reform in German cities, 1888–1912   179
10.3   The diffusion of infant welfare initiatives in German cities, 1888–1908   182

11.1   Infant mortality in Prussia 1877–1913   198
11.2   Acute digestive diseases: mortality 1877–1913 in German towns   202
11.3   Seasonal distribution of infant mortality in selected cities, 1898–1902   202
11.4   Seasonal distribution of infant mortality in Berlin (1908) according to feeding practices   204

11.5   Seasonal distribution of infant mortality in selected cities,
       1926–28   204
11.6   Infant mortality Regierungsbezirk Düsseldorf 1902–6   207

List of tables

9.1   Mortality, housing and population in a sample of 36
      towns in England and Wales in 1871   149
9.2   The public health share of local authority investment   150
9.3   Changes in living standards, public health expenditures
      and mortality 1783–1913   154
9.4   The contribution of changes in population densities, food
      and sanitation to the decline of mortality   159
9.5   The contribution of economic changes to the decline of
      mortality   162

10.1 Influences of sanitary conditions on enteric fever and
      diarrhoea   177
10.2 Sanitary conditions of housing in urban Germany c. 1900   178
10.3 Descriptive statistics of variables used in the analysis   185
10.4 The statistical analysis of the decline in infant mortality,
      1889–1912   186
10.5 The statistical analysis of the decline in infant mortality
      from diarrhoeal and other causes, 1903–12   187
10.6 Predicted impacts of changes in important variables on
      infant mortality   190

11.1 Cause-specific mortality changes in the largest German
      towns   197

Notes on contributors

Frances Bell was a research assistant until 1999 in the Department of History at the University of Manchester, financed by the Leverhulme Trust. She was awarded an MPhil with Distinction by Lancaster University in 1995 for her thesis on public health and mortality in nineteenth-century Preston.

John C. Brown is Associate Professor of Economics at Clark University in Massachusetts, USA. His research has focused on the economics of public health and he is currently researching the role of public health and other influences on the demography of German cities before the First World War. Publications include 'Comment: Science, Health and Household Technology: the effect of the Pasteur revolution', in Timothy F. Bresnahan and Robert J. Gordon (eds), *The Economics of New Goods* (Chicago, 1997).

Peter Christensen is an Assistant Professor in the Department of History at the University of Copenhagen. His research interests include comparative environmental history and the changing patterns of infectious diseases. Recent publications include *The decline of Iranshahr: irrigation and environments in the history of the Middle East 500BC to AD1500* (Copenhagen, 1993) and 'Middle Eastern irrigation: legacies and lessons', *Yale School of Forestry and Environmental Studies*, 103 (1998) 15–30.

Flurin Condrau is a temporary Senior Lecturer in the Department of Economic and Social History at the University of Munich. He received his D Phil in 1999 for his thesis on the social history of tuberculosis in Britain and Germany during the late nineteenth and early twentieth centuries. This will be published in *Kritische Studien zur Geschichtswissenschaft* (Goettingen, 2000).

Silke Fehlemann is a Lecturer in Modern History at the University of Dusseldorf. Her research interests include the history of German social policy, gender studies and the social history of medicine.

Peregrine Horden is a Wellcome Trust Research Lecturer in the History of Medicine at Royal Holloway, University of London and is a Fellow of All Souls College, Oxford. He is the editor (with Richard Smith) of *The Locus of*

Care (London, 1998) and the co-author with Nicholas Purcell of *The Corrupting Sea: A Study of Mediterranean History* (Oxford, 1999).

Colin Jones is Professor of History at Warwick University. His research interests focus on French history, particularly from the seventeenth to the early nineteenth century. His most recent book (authored with Laurence Brockliss) is *The Medical World of Early Modern France* (Oxford, 1998). Other publications include *The Charitable Imperative* (1989) and the *Cambridge Illustrated History of France* (1993). He currently is working on the history of the mouth.

Gerry Kearns is a Lecturer in Geography at the University of Cambridge. His research interests include the history of public health ideologies and the historical geography of Irish identities. Recent publications include *Urbanising Britain: Essays on Class and Community in the Nineteenth Century* (edited with Charles Withers, Cambridge, 1991) and 'Tuberculosis and the medicalisation of English society, 1880–1920' in John Woodward and Robert Jutte (eds), *Coping with Sickness: Historical Aspects of Health Care in a European Perspective* (Sheffield, 1995).

Paul Laxton is a Lecturer in Geography at the University of Liverpool.

Robert Millward is Professor of Economic History in the Department of History at the University of Manchester. He has written extensively on the history and economics of the public sector in Britain. Recent publications include *Public and Private Ownership of British Industry 1820–1990* (Oxford, 1994) and *The Political Economy of Nationalisation in Britain 1920–1950* (Cambridge, 1995). He also has joint authorship with Frances Bell of articles on the subject of public health in *Continuity and Change* (July 1998) and the *European Review of Economic History* (1998).

Marjaana Niemi is a researcher in the Department of History, University of Tampere, Finland. She completed her PhD at the University of Leicester, 'Health Experts and the Politics of Knowledge. Britain and Sweden, 1900–1940'. Her publications include 'Challenging authorities' views: women and health in British and Swedish cities, 1900–1920', in Marjatta Hietala and Lars Nilsson (eds), *Women in Towns* (1999). Her current research is on urban renewal in old industrial cities after the Second World War.

Helen Power is Wellcome Lecturer in the History of Medicine at the University of Liverpool. She has recently published *Tropical Medicine in the Twentieth Century: A History of the Liverpool School of Tropical Medicine,*

1889–1990 (London, 1999). Her research interests include public health and medical research in colonial India and Africa, particularly the history of malaria and drugs associated with its control.

Sally Sheard is Lecturer in the History of Public Health in the Department of Public Health and the School of History at the University of Liverpool. Her research interests include the political economy of public health and local government. Recent publications include 'Profit is a Dirty Word: the Development of Public Baths and Wash-houses in Britain 1847–1915, *Social History of Medicine*, 13.1 (2000), 63–85; and (with Chris Hamlin) 'Revolutions in Public Health: 1848 and 1998?' *British Medical Journal*, 317 (1998), 587–91.

Jakob Tanner is Professor of Modern History at the Research Institute for Social and Economic History at Zurich University, Switzerland. His research interests include the social and economic history of Europe and Switzerland, the history of the body and studies of science and technology. Recent publications include *Fabrikmahlzeit, Ernahrungswissenschaft, Industriearbiet und Volksernahrung in der Schweiz 1890–1950* (Zurich, 1999); 'The rationing system, food policy and nutritional science during the Second World War: a comparative view of Switzerland' in Carola Lentz (ed.), *Changing Food Habits. Case Studies from Africa, South America and Europe* (Australia USW, 1999).

Jorg Vogele is Assistant Director of the Institute for the History of Medicine at the University of Dusseldorf, Germany and Fellow of the School of History, University of Liverpool. His research interests are the demographic, economic and social history of England and Germany. He has recently published *Urban Mortality Change in England and Germany, 1870–1910* (Liverpool, 1998).

Wolfgang Woelk is a Lecturer in the Institute for the History of Medicine at the University of Dusseldorf, Germany. His research interests include the social, political and regional history of Germany. He co-edited *Die Medizinische Akademie Dusseldorf im Nationalsozialismus* (Essen, 1997).

Acknowledgements

Special thanks are due to Richard Rodger (as editor for the Historical Urban Studies series) and the various colleagues who have commented on the essays and assisted with the preparation of the volume. We also gratefully acknowledge the support and encouragement received from Jon Sheard and Bill Bynum.

Historical Urban Studies
general editors' preface

Density and proximity of buildings and people are two of the defining characteristics of the urban dimension. It is these which identify a place as uniquely urban, though the threshold for such pressure points varies from place to place. What is considered an important cluster in one context, may not be considered as urban elsewhere. A third defining characteristic is functionality – the commercial or strategic position of a town or city which conveys an advantage. Over time, these functional advantages may diminish, or the balance of advantage may change within a hierarchy of towns. To understand how the relative importance of towns shifts over time and space is to grasp a set of relationships which is fundamental to the study of urban history.

Towns and cities are products of history, yet have themselves helped to shape history. As the proportion of urban dwellers has increased, so the urban dimension has proved a legitimate unit of analysis through which to understand the spectrum of human experience and to explore the cumulative memory of past generations. Though obscured by layers of economic, social and political change, the study of the urban milieu provides insights into the functioning of human relationships and, if urban historians are not themselves directly concerned with current policy studies, few contemporary concerns can be understood without reference to the historical development of towns and cities.

This longer historical perspective is essential to an understanding of social processes. Crime, housing conditions and property values, health and education, discrimination and deviance, and the formulation of regulations and social policies to deal with them were, and remain, amongst the perennial preoccupations of towns and cities – no historical period has a monopoly of these concerns. They recur in successive generations, albeit in varying mixtures and strengths; the details may differ but the central forces of class, power and authority in the city remain. If this was the case for different periods, so it was for different geographical entities and cultures. Both scientific knowledge and technical information were available across Europe and showed little respect for frontiers. Yet despite common concerns and access to broadly similar knowledge, different solutions to urban problems were proposed and adopted by towns and cities in different parts of Europe. This comparative dimension informs urban historians as to which were systematic factors and which were of a purely local nature: general and particular forces can be distinguished.

These analytical frameworks, considered in a comparative context, inform the books in this series.

Jean-Luc Pinol
Richard Rodger

Centre de Recherches Historique sur la ville, Strasbourg
University of Leicester

Preface

This volume originated in a conference *Health in the City: A History of Public Health*, which was held in Liverpool in September 1997 under the aegis of the Society for the Social History of Medicine and the International Network for the History of Public Health. All of the essays in this volume were presented as conference papers, with the exception of the review essay by Sally Sheard and Helen Power, and the chapter by Colin Jones. The conference formed part of the wider celebrations in Liverpool in 1997 to mark the 150th anniversary of the appointment in 1847 of Britain's first Medical Officer of Health, Dr William Henry Duncan. Liverpool in the nineteenth century was alternately despised as the filthiest town in Britain and heralded as the champion of public health reform. Such a dual identity continues in many parts of life on Merseyside in the twenty-first century. The timing of the conference was also choice – coming shortly after the appointment in May 1997 of Britain's first government Minister for Public Health, Tessa Jowell MP. This renewed recognition of the importance of public health was reinforced by the publication of a government White Paper. These developments served as a reminder that both history and community health are live issues.

The location of the conference in Liverpool brought out some excellent 'local history' but also attracted participants and papers from around the globe. Despite the high standard of many of the non-European papers, we decided to concentrate on Europe. The essays in this volume are written from a range of very different disciplinary perspectives – geographers and demographers wearing historical hats, historians of medicine, administration, politics and religion. We have arranged the essays chronologically, yet do not claim to provide a comprehensive history of urban public health. These essays are examples of some of the most innovative research using a variety of methodologies, including biography, economic modelling and textual analysis.

There are some unifying themes within the volume – choice and contingency, control over the behaviour of individuals and communities, the interpretation of language and forms of communication. The importance of urban space as a special socio-political unit is not a new concept, but considering the health of the city in terms of the language, symbols and discourse of public health enriches this tradition. Links between the disciplines of medical history and urban history and, indeed, between the individual essays in this volume, are found in the notion of space both as a physical area and as a community. An equally significant theme is that of the languages of disease and health, in particular the use of language in the negotiation of space and community. In such a movement towards a greater understanding of health in the city, consideration must also be given to the people who occupy the space within the city, who are themselves part of the definition of that area as a social, political and cultural space. Moreover, the concept of space is not limited to defining traditional boundaries negotiated through maps; space may also be usefully employed in an interpretation of the individual body – sick, polluting, healthy or in need of protection – and in the identification of the collective body of community health.

1

Body and city: medical and urban histories of public health

Sally Sheard and Helen Power

What is it about urban life that has historically given it an unhealthy reputation – an image that continues to persist into the twenty-first century in many countries and cultures? For urban-dwellers and those who have sought to describe their experiences there has been an enduring interest in the relationship between urban life and health. Within the earliest cities there was a tacit recognition that urbanisation could only be sustained through the adoption of a set of guidelines for 'living in proximity by consent'. In some places this was formalised through specific ordinances, in others it can be seen in the cultural assumptions about what constituted a 'healthy lifestyle'. Yet the substructure to many of these discourses is that urban health has often been inherently poor for the majority of urban-dwellers. From the biblical cities onwards, commentators have sought to identify the evils of urban life as symbols of man's estrangement from God, the theatre of man's spiritual degeneration.[1] Within this genre, Babylon is portrayed by the prophets as representative of the evils of all cities of the world and, later, Augustine uses the example of Rome in *City of God* as proof of the frailty of all things human.[2] Health, or more specifically the absence of health and the 'visitation' of disease, become spiritual and practical indicators of the problems and deficiencies of urban life.

The diseased city

Epidemic infectious disease in particular exposes the weaknesses in urban communities, highlights the disparities in income and associated living conditions that accompany urbanisation. It facilitates recognition that shared residency and limited citizenship do not necessarily guarantee a genuine moral

---

[1]   A. Lees, *Cities Perceived: Urban Society in European and American Thought, 1820–1940* (Manchester, 1985), p. 6.
[2]   Ibid., p. 7.

or cultural community. Urban public health has been sought – and sometimes achieved – through a myriad of political, social, economic and medical strategies. Many of them have been direct responses to the threat of specific infectious diseases. Such reactive measures were usually aimed at ensuring the immediate health of the public and were not usually articulated as part of a cumulative, 'improving' crusade. However, the chronic fear of infectious disease, which impregnated all urban centres from the early modern period onwards, resulted in an inherited knowledge of control strategies which could be rekindled when required. Thus the imminent arrival of plague in medieval European cities in 1348, after an absence of some five centuries, triggered dormant quarantine and disinfection procedures. The recurring epidemics – every six to thirteen years until the mid-sixteenth century and then again in the late seventeenth century – ensured that urban authorities always had a core knowledge of how to cope with plague epidemics.

The first three essays in this volume were selected for the insight they provide into pre-modern urban responses to threats to the public's health. Peregrine Horden focuses on the rituals which were stimulated by diseases such as plague in the early medieval urban centres of Europe. Much of the rich documentation which survives from this period of urban history comes from religious sources. Through a specifically health-based interpretation of the texts of the first-century Bishop Gregory of Tours – who was well acquainted with the tradition of religious men serving their communities as all-purpose public authorities and urban administrators – Horden is able to illustrate that they provided the 'attentive' with models for both collective and individual action in averting future epidemics. They reassert the maxim that health is spiritual, social, not simplistically medical. The ritual procedures which Horden deconstructs – the separation of the sacred and the diseased, vigilance, penitentials in the face of threatened social dislocation – demonstrate not a miraculous power in the biblical sense, but certain 'techniques' for the reconfiguration of urban space to minimise the impact of disease in the urban area. These techniques were managed by a style of urban leadership which is comparable with the vigour and comprehensiveness of the later Health Boards of the Renaissance.[3]

Horden's essay also makes a valuable contribution to our knowledge of urban health initiatives in those non-epidemic periods which have proved so elusive for the historian. However, his most significant suggestion is this: by adding a religious dimension to the established account of the origins of modern social hygiene it is possible to flesh out the bare narratives which currently occupy the period between the Roman empire and the Italian city-

---

[3]   See C.M. Cipolla, *Miasmas and Disease. Public Health and the Environment in the Pre-Industrial Age* (New Haven and London, 1992).

states of the Renaissance. Recognition of the significance of urban pollution and hygiene by urban authorities and the urban public can be observed within the ritual language of penitentials, not just within the traditionalist narrow confines of the early Middle Ages, but also located in Jewish, Roman, Frankish and Venetian cultures with sufficient substance to permit a reinterpretation of the evolution of modern social hygiene.[4]

Colin Jones uses his essay to raise awareness of the problems associated with using accounts of plague. He suggests that historians need to use caution when interpreting texts at face value. On one level, these sources may tell us basic facts about the disease, but Jones argues that they would be of more interest if they were used to look at the impact of disease on society. There are, according to Jones, three 'scripts' within many of the plague treatises, which operate with similar symbolic systems based on the metaphor of the body violated by plague. Thus the medical script is focused on the patient, the religious script on the loss of spiritual 'body' as Christian community. The third script is administrative or political and addressed to the citizen – articulating the fear of social and economic dislocation brought about in times of epidemic disease and resulting in the institution of anti-plague measures. Jones reminds us that it is within the city – a particular space and community – that the administrative actions found in the texts are made manifest. We can read the texts as a window onto past experiences of the plague, as suffered at these three overlapping levels. But as Jones's interest is in a questioning of the 'literary character' and 'rhetorical purposes' of these texts, he suggests that they may have been intended to serve purposes other than composite pictures of the plague experience so far revealed. What we need, he urges, is a print history of plague texts, which would raise a new set of questions so far unasked by historians, despite the extensive historiography. He concludes this challenging essay with reference to the symbolic effects of plague, the language used to create such effects and their wider social and cultural resonance. What is significant is the acknowledgement that it is the experience of plague which has informed many of the subsequent attitudes to other urban infectious diseases, particularly cholera.

An example of what one might classify as an 'administrative script' is found in the next essay. The location is eighteenth-century Denmark, and Peter Christensen delivers a narrative which enhances existing accounts of plague in Europe. The circumstances of the 1711 epidemic, arriving in the midst of the Great Northern War, illuminate the additional stress which epidemic disease placed on urban authorities. The early cases of plague in Copenhagen were

---

[4]   These themes are also developed in R. Sennett, *Flesh and Stone: The Body and the City in Western Civilisation* (London, 1996). This builds on the work of Mary Douglas and the Chicago School of urban sociology in investigating the ways in which 'urban spaces take form largely from the ways in which people experience their own bodies' (p. 370).

ignored by the authorities, whose delayed response, Christensen suggests, was due to the economic implications of declaring a quarantine. This theme is echoed by a later essay in this volume by Gerry Kearns, who finds a similar quandary facing Liverpool's Medical Officer of Health during a cholera epidemic. It is interesting that after the plague had subsided in Copenhagen, complaints were made about the activities of the specially appointed Health Commission. Some accused the Commission of inefficiency, others suggested it had been too 'high-handed'. What is evident is that when the traditional protections such as quarantine failed, the city lacked a clear sense of management.

The nineteenth-century urban revolution

The enduring negative images of urban areas which persisted through the Enlightenment were in part based on analyses of urban health conditions. In England John Graunt and William Petty's statistical investigations fuelled fears that high urban mortality rates were unsustainable and that urbanisation was sapping the true wealth of the country – its population. On the Continent the potentially damaging nature of urbanisation was used by Rousseau in his novel *Emile*, which portrayed Paris as a 'moloch' feeding greedily on the blood of provincial Frenchmen, corrupting those that it did not kill.[5] However, it was the nineteenth century which experienced the most dramatic changes in urban life. In 1800 London was the only Western city to have passed the million mark (Paris had a population of 547,000, Berlin 172,000, New York 60,000). By 1940 there were nineteen other cities with over a million inhabitants. Yet the most fascinating feature of urbanisation during this period is the changes it brought to urban areas of all sizes.

Is it necessary to define 'urban'? Perhaps a more significant question would be: do we need a definition for the purposes of a history of urban public health? There are two common approaches to defining 'urban' – both of which have implications for the essays in this volume. The first approach is exemplified by C.M. Law, who used a population threshold approach to his classic study of urbanisation in nineteenth-century England and Wales.[6] Urban size has had significant implications for public health. Research has shown that expectations

---

[5]   J.J. Rousseau, *Emile* (Paris, 1762).
[6]   C.M. Law, 'The Growth of Urban Population in England and Wales, 1801–1911', *Transactions of the Institute of British Geographers*, 41 (1967), 125–43.

of health and life decreased with increasing urban size during the nineteenth century.[7] Woods has expressed this in a most vivid way:

> A male baby born in an inner area of Liverpool in 1861 could be expected to live 26 years whilst a female might be expected to live an additional year. In Okehampton, Devon, comparable life expectations would have been 57 years and 55 years for males and females respectively.[8]

This was a pattern common to many European countries. Yet it is not urban size *per se* which is important, but the conditions within the urban area, and this brings us to our second way of defining 'urban'. By approaching the concept of the 'urban' through 'urbanism', which suggests a particular and distinctive urban way of life we can begin to interpret the political, economic and social circumstances which made life in urban areas so different. Urban places usually had traditions of market culture and well-identified managerial institutions. As centres of commerce, with associated high land values, they could afford through a rating system to pay for a more 'cultivated' way of life – street paving, civic buildings and communal facilities such as water supplies.[9]

Histories of cities have been written from a number of perspectives. Some fall into a group which is exemplified by the work of Philip Abrams, which tend to ignore the existence of the city as an independent social reality. Richard Dennis makes this summary of the Abrams style of history: 'Towns should be treated as battles rather than monuments, a dynamic perspective reminiscent of E.P. Thompson's treatment of classes as happenings, not things'.[10] A second approach, although perhaps not an outright contradiction of the Abrams mode of analysis, is seen in the work of the classic urban historian Jim Dyos, who concentrated his research quite specifically on the problems of cities, using local studies.[11] Research which explicitly views the city as a political arena has almost inevitably been generated from the preoccupations with class and conflict in an urban context. Gerry Kearns and Charles Withers provide a

---

[7]   G. Kearns, 'The Urban Penalty and the Population History of England', in A. Brandstrom and L.-G. Tedebrand (eds), *Society, Health and Population During the Demographic Transition* (Stockholm, 1988), pp. 213–38.

[8]   R. Woods, 'Mortality Patterns in the Nineteenth Century', in R. Woods and J. Woodward (eds), *Urban Disease and Mortality In Nineteenth Century England* (London, 1984), p. 40.

[9]   For a useful overview of nineteenth-century British urbanisation see R.J. Morris and R. Rodger, 'An Introduction to British Urban History 1920–1914', in R.J. Morris and R. Rodger (eds), *The Victorian City 1820–1914* (Leicester, 1993), pp. 1–39.

[10]   R. Dennis, *English Industrial Cities of the Nineteenth Century: a Social Geography* (Cambridge, 1984) p. 290.

[11]   H.J. Dyos, *The Study of Urban History* (London, 1968); H.J. Dyos and M. Wolff, *The Victorian City* (London, 1973). See also D. Cannadine and D. Reeder (eds), *Exploring the Urban Past: Essays in Urban History by H.J. Dyos* (Cambridge, 1982).

useful digest in the introduction to their edited volume, which neatly analyses the recent historiography.[12] Kearns's own essay within that volume is an excellent examination of the way in which class 'permeated the reality of the biological basis of society but also promoted a biological view of social and political relations', and it anticipates some of the more recent developments in medical urban history.[13]

Yet the speed of urbanisation, stimulated (first in Britain and then later in Europe) by industrialisation, was not matched by a transformation in urban management. The existing institutions – corporations, councils, improvement commissions – could not keep pace with the changes. New urban housing was constructed to meet market demand, without consideration for overcrowding. There was little attempt at town planning and the provision of basic sanitary services was non-existent in many places.[14] Thus, rapid urbanisation was accompanied by a deterioration in the condition of the urban environment. Having broken the fundamental principle of 'living in proximity by consent', the consequence was an increase in pollution, infectious diseases moving from endemic to epidemic proportions and a general decrease in urban life expectancy. Up to a point, the mechanics of urbanisation, involving mass in-migration from rural areas, can disguise the demographic imbalance caused by high mortality rates. However, there comes a moment when a critical threshold is reached, and the hitherto accepted conditions of urban life are called sharply into question.

In Britain, the problems of urbanisation were articulated most convincingly through the cholera and typhus epidemics of the 1830s and 1840s. They provoked a reassessment of the mechanics of urban management, and recognised the need for a proactive public health ideology. Liverpool might have been the first town to adopt a public health policy, but it was only a few steps ahead of national legislation.[15] However, this first national Public Health Act, passed in 1848, was fundamentally flawed. Its permissive nature and the piecemeal pattern of creation of local boards of health reflected the strong defence of local government autonomy and the public's perception of the role of urban management. As Chris Hamlin has shown, concepts of what public health entailed in mid-Victorian Britain were very different from our current

---

[12]   G. Kearns and C.W.J. Withers (eds), *Urbanising Britain. Essays on Class and Community in the Nineteenth Century* (Cambridge, 1991).

[13]   Ibid., p. 9; G. Kearns, 'Biology, Class and the Urban Penalty', pp. 12–30.

[14]   See A.S. Wohl, *Endangered Lives. Public Health in Victorian Britain* (London, 1984), for some of the best descriptions of the evils of unplanned urban growth.

[15]   C. Hamlin and S. Sheard, 'Revolutions in Public Health: 1848 and 1998?', *British Medical Journal*, 317 (1998), 587–91.

interpretations.[16] For the first half of the nineteenth century the terms 'sanitary reform' and 'public health' were almost interchangeable. The medical–public health marriage had yet to be formalised, and the practical solutions of the civil engineers were triumphant. Hamlin expertly identifies the ways in which Chadwick's 'sanitarianism' fitted the political needs of the Poor Law and the governments of the day and the ensuing problems of placing responsibility for reform with local and central government. Yet by making the system, rather than the reformer, the focus of analysis, Hamlin is able to progress the recent historiography of public health and distance it from the Whiggish 'heroic' accounts so ably presented by R.A. Lewis, S.E. Finer and others.[17] It is also important to remember that countries have not always needed the stimuli of industrialisation to introduce public health policies. The wide range of experiences assembled for Dorothy Porter's edited volume *The History of Public Health and the Modern State* stress the diversity of public health interventions – from Sweden in the eighteenth century through to the system of medical police developed by Johann Peter Frank in Prussia.[18] These philosophies pre-date the explosion of European urbanisation of the nineteenth century, but find common ground in the recognition of the need for urban health professionals and the cultivation of individual responsibility for the collective health of the urban community.

The essays by Paul Laxton and Gerry Kearns focus on one of the first public health professionals – Dr William Henry Duncan – and on mid-nineteenth-century Liverpool, probably one of the most notorious towns in the context of urban public health. Liverpool featured extensively in the investigations of Edwin Chadwick into the relationship between urban growth and mortality in the 1830s and 1840s. There are two reasons for its prominence. First, it was one of the most unhealthy towns in Britain – identified in a Registrar-General's report as 'the Black spot on the Mersey' – second, it had gained recognition for its pioneering sanitary reforms of the 1840s. Laxton's detailed study of Duncan's activities after his appointment as Liverpool's Medical Officer of Health in 1847 (the first such post in Britain) illustrates the benefits to be gained from a rejuvenation of the discipline of biography in the study of history of medicine. The advantages of examining public health practitioners within their social context and relating their changing ideas and practices to a larger structure of political and economic conditions were highlighted by George Rosen, undoubtedly one of the most respected public health historians of the

---

[16]   C. Hamlin, *Public Health and Social Justice in the Age of Chadwick, 1800–1854* (Cambridge, 1998). The introduction provides an excellent analysis of the definitions of 'public health'.

[17]   R.A. Lewis, *Edwin Chadwick and the Public Health Movement, 1832–1854* (London, 1952); S.E. Finer, *The Life and Times of Edwin Chadwick* (London, 1952).

[18]   D. Porter (ed.), *The History of Public Health and the Modern State* (Amsterdam, 1994).

twentieth century.[19] More recently, Ludmilla Jordanova has argued that medical history may be enhanced through the non-direct appropriation of knowledge about medical practices and institutions and for a re-evaluation of the medical-biographical tool.[20] Laxton is able to illustrate the various social and economic pressures suffered by Duncan in his campaigns to improve the health of Liverpool. The heavily environmentalist slant of Duncan's strategies provides an excellent practical example of the preoccupations of Chadwick and public health engineers with 'cleaning up' the towns. Additionally, these policies, where they came into open conflict with property interests, show the relative strength (or perhaps weakness) of health as a political tool and as an indicator of public recognition of the threat of disease. Laxton develops examples in his essay which illustrate clearly the importance of urban form and geographical segregation for health issues. In 1847 during a typhus epidemic, Duncan requests that fever sheds – temporary accommodation for fever patients – are erected in an upper-class residential area, favoured for its 'healthy' environment. The Medical Officer of Health's determination to put a potential source of infection within this influential community caused outrage. Representations to the urban authorities reflected on the loss of value to property as well as the threat of contracting typhus. Duncan was isolated in his battle, in which his epidemiological evidence could not match the economic strength of the residents and their political spokespersons. Laxton's analysis is a welcome asset in the reinterpretation of nineteenth-century public health reform. A number of historians have already made the case for divorcing public health history from its Whiggish pedigree. However, its reconstruction requires local studies of this type, which show the complexities of public health in an urban context, acknowledging its part in an integrated system alongside property development and the formation of class-based urban pressure groups.

Gerry Kearns's essay builds on the valuable biography of Dr William Henry Duncan provided by Paul Laxton, and uses the Liverpool example to investigate the interplay between central and local government in the formation of public health policy in nineteenth-century Britain. In acknowledging the role of the Medical Officer of Health as a mediator in medico-political disputes, such as the contagion versus anti-contagion debate, he facilitates a more subtle investigation of health professionals within the urban context. Thus, Duncan's declaration of an epidemic in Liverpool becomes a political statement rather than a straightforward medical observance, made with full cognisance of the economic implications which his professional comment would have on the trade of the port. Kearns elaborates his hypothesis through a dissection of the

---

[19]   E. Fee, 'Public Health Past and Present', in G. Rosen, *A History of Public Health* (expanded edn, 1993), p. x.
[20]   L. Jordanova, 'The Social Construction of Medical Knowledge', *Social History of Medicine*, 7 (1995), 361–81.

interaction between principles and practices in disease reporting, identifying specifically commercial as well as medical principles. For Kearns, Duncan seems to be a more positive figure than he is for Laxton. Duncan appears to control his situation, carefully choosing his strategies for public information according to his audience. In the campaign for the local Sanatory Act in 1846 he uses the rhetoric of shame over Liverpool's high mortality rates. After the Act is achieved (but before the essential sanitary reform expenditure has been agreed) he switches to an appeal to the Town Council's sense of 'civic pride'. This is reminiscent of the contrasting pessimistic/optimistic views of other mid-nineteenth-century urban commentators such as Thomas Chalmers and Robert Vaughan. Vaughan had a subtitle for his 1841 book, *The Age of Great Cities: Modern Civilisation Viewed in Relation to Intelligence, Morals and Religion*. This would probably have found favour with Duncan, for whom urbanisation was not merely an economic phenomenon, but a reflection of society and culture, and a primary determinant of health experiences.

Public health as political expediency

If the essays by Paul Laxton and Gerry Kearns help to illustrate the early 'sanitary era' and the formation of basic principles of urban public health management, the following essay shows how fledgling sanitary reform systems could be thrown into disarray by epidemic disease. Flurin Condrau and Jacob Tanner continue the analysis of specific diseases within an urban context. Their analysis of the public's response to cholera in Zurich in 1867 illustrates the universal fear associated with epidemic disease which also features in Peter Christensen's investigation of Copenhagen's plague epidemics. Yet it is interesting to observe the impact of nineteenth-century industrialisation and urbanisation through the experience of Zurich. Condrau and Tanner show, through carefully selected anecdotes, that the public's perception of infectious epidemics had not changed significantly from earlier centuries – there was still the abandonment of public social interactions and the use of amulets to give protection. However, within the unsettled political situation in Zurich the cholera epidemic was loaded with metaphors and seen as an expression of the ailing democratic system. This 1867 epidemic pushed beyond the reactive quarantine measures and posited a practical, sanitary solution to socio-economic difficulties as expressed through epidemic infectious disease. Condrau and Tanner identify the persistence of some elements of the miasmatic theory into the final decades of the nineteenth century (after the developments of germ theory) with a political application: it enabled the linkage of sick bodies to a sick system and helped to model the semantics of urban political reform. More explicitly, they recognise the adoption of specific urban–rural contrasts in the application of certain antonyms to urban health polemics: musty vs. fresh, spoiled vs. pure, artificial vs. natural, dirty vs. clean, dark vs. light. The relationship between urbanisation and health, as articulated through an epidemic, differs markedly from that described by Christensen, and also from the earlier accounts provided by Horden. Condrau and Tanner's investigation clearly shows how the integrated political, economic and social structures of urban areas by the mid-nineteenth century changed and were changed by health conditions, specifically epidemic disease. Their recognition of the importance of the attitudes of urban health authorities and their integration into the urban political system echoes similar themes in the essays by Marjaana Niemi, Paul Laxton and Gerry Kearns, for whom the focus on the public health professional is a useful tool in analysing urban public health histories.

Marjaana Niemi's essay is a valuable exponent of interdisciplinary studies of urban public health, showing an awareness of the political economy of early twentieth-century public health strategies in an explicitly geographical context. Her comparative analysis of Birmingham and Gothenburg at the end of the nineteenth century and into the first decades of the twentieth century considers the political and scientific justification for the differing styles of public health analysis and policy, specifically in the mapping of urban health problems and the development of tuberculosis strategies. The focus of the Medical Officer of Health for Birmingham on insanitary areas, articulated through maps which showed large parts of the urban centre ominously shaded in black, contrasts with the approach in Gothenburg which identified individual 'unhealthy' houses. These initial statistical analyses supported very different public health strategies. For example, in Birmingham health visitors were sent into all homes within designated 'unhealthy' areas, whereas in Gothenburg resources were targeted more precisely – health visitors only called on specific families and those with newborn babies which were not being breastfed. At first glance, it would appear that Gothenburg operated a more sophisticated public health system. Yet Niemi suggests that we must observe a more fundamental process in operation than the superficial efficiency of a system. The Gothenburg approach reflects the selections made by the health authorities from a wide range of 'scientific' information, available internationally by the end of the nineteenth century, on such complex issues as the mode of transmission of tuberculosis. These choices were dependent upon the power of the health authorities in local political systems. Thus in Gothenburg, although tuberculosis was primarily seen as a 'dwelling disease', there was no political support for large-scale investment in public housing to improve living conditions, and tuberculosis patients were instead hospitalised. These control measures were directly allied to medical paternalism. In Birmingham such individualistic medical strategies could not compete with the entrenched environmentalist dogma, which preached health education on unhealthy behaviour. Niemi's essay connects with wider discourses on the implications of socio-economic segregation in urban areas by the late nineteenth century. By comparing Birmingham (a typical British city) which experienced substantial residential segregation early in the century in addition to large-scale suburban growth, with Gothenburg, which despite population growth maintained a compact and relatively unsegregated urban core, we can begin to see how health issues were manipulated geographically to advance particular political agendas. Thus, in Gothenburg the notion of healthy and unhealthy areas was not an important conceptual tool in explaining urban health problems.

Public health within the new urban history horoscope

Gerry Kearns uses his essay to make the important point that studies of urban public health must acknowledge the distinctive political cultures both of Whitehall and of individual town halls. This reinforces the work of Derek Fraser, Peter Hennock and others on the development of municipal government in nineteenth-century Britain.[21] This cluster of urban history research was undertaken in the 1970s and 1980s and, as has been noted elsewhere, can be interpreted as symptomatic of the wider dissatisfaction with life in urban Britain at this time. Some of the historians within this genre are happy to act as narrators, and as such provide interesting synopses. See, for example, Sidney Checkland's 'Urban History Horoscope' in Derek Fraser and Anthony Sutcliffe's edited volume, *The Pursuit of Urban History*.[22] Checkland dissects the thematic agendas and he attributes the domination of certain themes, the social for example, to the way in which particular disciplines have developed within the social sciences. Thus the boom in sociology in the 1960s and 1970s produced a cohort of publications on urban social history. At the time of writing in 1985, Checkland's third and fourth themes for urban history – political process and economics – were still thin.[23] The subsequent monograph by David Harvey, *The Urbanisation of Capital*, provided fresh ideas on the centrality of the urban experience to political and economic processes as well as social and spatial structures.[24] Medical urban history has also had its share of reviews and discussions, many of which have highlighted the failure of these separate avenues of research to converge. Bill Luckin's seminal review 'Death

---

[21]   D. Fraser, Municipal Reform and the Industrial City (Leicester, 1982); *idem, Power and Authority in the Victorian City* (Oxford, 1983); E.P. Hennock, *Fit and Proper Persons* (London, 1973).

[22]   S. Checkland, 'An Urban History Horoscope', in D. Fraser and A. Sutcliffe (eds), *The Pursuit of Urban History* (1983), pp. 449–66.

[23]   Ibid., p. 453.

[24]   D. Harvey, *The Urbanisation of Capital* (Oxford, 1985).

and survival in the city: approaches to the history of disease', was published in the *Urban History Yearbook* in 1980, yet it contains many provocative suggestions which have still not been fully taken up by either urban or medical historians.[25]

Wealth, particularly its expression through property, has always been central to the development of public health policy. First, the cost of sanitary programmes, such as the installation of water supplies, sewerage systems and street paving, could not be met without a local taxation system based on property values. Second, sanitary reform ultimately required access to and the rights to interfere with what Gerry Kearns has elsewhere labelled the 'sanctity of property'.[26] Kearns suggests that the arguments for the nineteenth-century British environmentalist public health policies were constructed with great sensitivity to the paradox – they would only work if public health problems could be made to relate to market failures such as water supply and housing – 'thereby conceding that there were some areas of the economy where the market could not be trusted to hold sway'.[27] Achieving this concession was only part of the battle fought by urban public health reformers. To begin with, these reformers were not united, either geographically or ideologically. Hamlin has investigated the 'pipes and sewers wars' and more recently disentangled the varied ambitions of Edwin Chadwick to highlight the personal financial gains which Chadwick pursued through his integrated sewer system enterprise.[28] Raising the required capital was often just as difficult as choosing and designing the systems. The cost of sanitary reform was borne entirely locally, by property owners who were already rated for Poor Law and other local services. The rating system was especially onerous for the middle classes, who invested heavily in property. Despite their representation in local government, their control over levels of investment slipped away during the century as central government imposed more precise definitions of sanitary reform through compulsory legislation. The unprecedented levels of investment made by urban authorities in the 1880s and 1890s in public health infrastructure

---

[25]   W. Luckin, 'Death and survival in the city: approaches to the history of disease', *Urban History Yearbook* (1980), 53–62. See also review essays in other urban history journals: M. Fissell, 'Health in the city: putting together the pieces', *Urban History*, 19 (1992), 251–6; M Dupree, 'Medicine Comes to Town: Medicine and Social Structure in Urban Britain 1780–1870', *Journal of Urban History*, 17 (1990), 79–83.

[26]   G. Kearns, 'Private Property and Public Health Reform in England, 1830–1870', *Social Science and Medicine*, 24 (1987), 187–99.

[27]   Ibid., p. 187.

[28]   C. Hamlin, 'Muddling in Bumbledom: On the Enormity of Large Sanitary Improvements in Four British Towns, 1855–1885', *Victorian Studies*, 32 (1980), 55–83; *idem*, 'Edwin Chadwick and the Engineers, 1842–1854: Systems and Anti-Systems in the Pipe and Brick Sewers War', *Technology and Culture*, 33 (1992), 680–709 ; *idem*, 'Public Health and Social Justice in the Age of Chadwick'.

pushed the tolerance of the propertied classes to breaking point.[29] As Dorothy Porter has argued, public health is neither the salvation of society nor an agent of total repression. It represents most often a rather more interesting ground between the two extremes, but for many countries it has been the tool for the expansion of authoritarian bureaucratic government.[30]

Nurturing numbers: the potential of statistical analysis for urban public health histories

The last three essays in this collection develop this theme of the political economy of public health investment, specifically its relationship with mortality. Robert Millward and Frances Bell use a sample of thirty-six towns and cities in England and Wales to investigate the timing and magnitude of investment in public health. They suggest that the idea of 'choice' in the development of urban environments is critical. By using a range of statistical analyses they are able to illustrate that some of the commonly-held preconceptions about sanitary reform – in particular the hypothesis that most towns installed public health infrastructures in the middle of the nineteenth century – need to be repositioned within public health chronology. This is doubly significant. First, it contributes to a more accurate picture of the complexities and stresses of urban life in Britain at the end of an intensive period of urbanisation. It thus enriches the research of Williamson and other urban economic historians such as Daunton.[31] Millward and Bell provide a model which successfully allows for a reinterpretation of the economic and political context in which urban governments made their decisions on public health expenditure – which was, after all, one of the main items in the largest category of capital investment in the period 1870–1914.[32] This goes some way to redressing the inherently negative analyses of nineteenth-century urban growth which have persisted through their association with respected urban

---

[29]   S. Sheard, 'Profit is a Dirty Word: the development of public baths and wash-houses in Britain, 1847–1915', *Social History of Medicine*, 13 (2000), 63–85. See also A. Offer, *Property and Politics, 1870–1914: Landownership, Law, Ideology and Urban Development in England* (Cambridge, 1981).

[30]   D. Porter, *Health, Civilisation and the State: a History of Public Health from Ancient to Modern Times* (London, 1999), pp. 1–8.

[31]   J. Williamson, *Coping with City Growth During the British Industrial Revolution* (Cambridge, 1990); M.J. Daunton, 'Health and Housing in Victorian London', *Medical History*, supplement no. 11 (1991), 126–44. It is important to acknowledge the significant technical achievements in nineteenth-century urban design which this investment facilitated. For examples see J.A. Tarr and G. Dupuy (eds), *Technology and the Rise of the Networked City* (Philadelphia, 1988).

[32]   R. Millward and S. Sheard, 'The urban fiscal problem, 1870–1914: government expenditure and finance in England and Wales', *Economic History Review*, 48.3 (1995), 505.

historians. See, for example, Lewis Mumford's generalisations in *The City in History*, which fail to appreciate the achievements of urban financial management, but play instead upon the popular image of the degraded urban area.[33] Millward and Bell identify the tremendous improvements made in urban infrastructure, drawing on an increasingly tight local property resource and directed in many places by financially naïve town councillors.

Second, the Millward and Bell essay also informs an ongoing debate within urban historical demography on the causes of mortality decline. Rosen initiated a long-running debate in the 1950s with the suggestion that the decline of some infectious diseases before their correct mode of transmission was understood was in some part due to the impact of the earlier sanitary reform movement.[34] However, it required the revisionist bravado of Thomas McKeown in 1976 to establish an alternative hypothesis.[35] McKeown's vowed intention – of proving how little medical advances had contributed to the improved health of mankind – spawned a lucrative line of research for historical demographers. Accounting for the decline in mortality from specific diseases, as well as the overall changes in the demographic structure of the Western world, provided ample work through the 1980s and 1990s. Much of this research has had an explicitly urban focus. This can be partly explained by the academic credentials of the researchers, many of whom were based in geography departments and who could manipulate their interests in urban spatial form to accommodate this new area of research. Projects developed along mutually beneficial paths, some focusing on the specific diseases which figured in the McKeown hypothesis (cholera, typhus, tuberculosis), while others pieced together urban mortality series.[36] By the 1990s increasingly sophisticated computer analyses and the development of geographical information systems (GIS) made it possible to trace the finer nuances of mortality patterns. The urban factor in the equation took on a new significance when the size of the 'urban penalty' was finally

---

[33]   L. Mumford, *The City in History* (London, 1961), p. 509.

[34]   Fee, 'Public Health Past and Present', p. xxx.

[35]   T. McKeown and R. G. Record, 'Reasons for the Decline in Mortality in England and Wales in the Nineteenth Century', *Population Studies*, 16 (1962), 94–122; T. McKeown, *The Modern Rise of Population* (London, 1976).

[36]   There is a vast amount of literature now in this area. Dorothy Porter provides a valuable bibliography in *Health, Civilisation and the State*. See in particular A. Hardy, *The Epidemic Streets. Infectious disease and the rise of preventive medicine, 1856–1900* (Oxford, 1993); G. Cronje, 'Tuberculosis and mortality decline in England and Wales 1851–1910', in R. Woods and J. Woodward (eds), *Urban Disease and Mortality in Nineteenth Century England* (London, 1984), pp. 79–101; and B. Luckin, 'Evaluating the Sanitary Revolution: Typhus and Typhoid in London 1851–1900', in Woods and Woodward, *Urban Disease and Mortality*, pp. 102–20. Important early attempts to deconstruct the McKeown hypothesis include R. Woods, 'Mortality Patterns in the Nineteenth Century', in Woods and Woodward, *Urban Disease and Mortality*, pp. 37–64; G. Kearns, 'The Urban Penalty and the Population History of England'.

reliably calculated.[37] Simon Szreter's seminal paper in *Social History of Medicine* thus received its eagerly-awaited statistical validation.[38]

The penultimate essay in this collection is by John Brown. With its theme of economics and infant mortality decline in German towns between 1889 and 1912, it complements the town-based economic modelling of Millward and Bell by providing a household-level analysis of behaviour and expenditure. It also supplements the following essay by Vogele, Woelk and Fehlemann which focuses on the same period in German urban history. Brown uses models of household behaviour to determine the relative influences on infant mortality. This essay is an exciting justification that there is more mileage in the post-Szreter mortality decline debate. It attempts a more advanced integration of economic decision-making into the modelling of urban health. Practically, this means that we can elaborate on the hypothesis posed by Vogele, Woelk and Fehlemann that urban milk dispensaries had a negligible impact on diarrhoeal mortality rates. Brown's analysis suggests that the improved conditions for raising infants which women who worked could achieve, with their enhanced family income, more than offset the disadvantage of having less time available to care for their infants. He also shows that breastfeeding made little difference to infant mortality – more important determinants were poverty (particularly of single mothers) and poor sanitary provision. This provides an interesting contradiction to the health education efforts described by Vogele, Woelk and Felhemann.

The central tenet of the essay by Jorg Vogele, Wolfgang Woelk and Silke Fehlemann is that recent research has undervalued the contribution made by public health measures to the reduction in urban mortality in Western European cities at the end of the nineteenth century. The German urban areas exhibited an earlier decline in mortality rates than that shown for Britain. However, the domination of gastrointestinal diseases in the 1870s and 1880s – which predominantly afflicted infants – directed the attention and resources of the urban health authorities towards initiatives such as milk supply and infant welfare centres. Yet problems such as the small quantity of treated milk available, and its high cost, reduced the impact this public health measure could have made on infant mortality. Vogele, Woelk and Fehlemann highlight the economic motivations for the increase in breastfeeding rates during the First World War and they suggest that this was more significant than the health education campaigns. Through their detailed study of the activities of the

---

[37]   R. Woods and N. Shelton, *An Atlas of Victorian Mortality* (Liverpool, 1997). See also B. Luckin and G. Mooney, 'Urban history and historical epidemiology: the case of London, 1860–1920', *Urban History* (1997), 37–55.

[38]   S. Szreter, 'The Importance of Social Intervention in Britain's Mortality Decline, 1850–1914: a Reinterpretation of the Role of Public Health', *Social History of Medicine*, 1 (1988), 1–37.

Society for Infant Welfare in the administrative district of Dusseldorf (founded in 1907), they indicate the gap in social welfare policy which had been created by the rapid pace of urbanisation in nineteenth-century Germany. The failure of large urban areas to quickly construct social support systems and viable local communities had found its expression in low levels of health-care knowledge. In addition, the opposition of local doctors to the Society's welfare centres (for fear of reducing their incomes) illustrates neatly the complexities and economic battles of urban healthcare. This investigation of how the Society prioritised its services, identified infants 'at risk' and calculated financial inducements to healthier lifestyles forms an essential counterpart to the statistical analyses performed by John Brown. Here are the minutiae of urban public health history without which we fail to approach our goal of a fully-integrated discipline.

Conclusion

This collection of essays makes no pretence at being a comprehensive account of the history of urban public health. There are considerable gaps in chronology and no discussion of non-European experiences. None of the essays discuss events after the 1920s. Yet, to some extent, this is a natural point at which to break the long narrative of urban health. By this date several European countries had reached their saturation point for urbanisation. For example, Britain had 78 per cent of its population living in urban areas by 1911.[39] The urban variable had declined in importance by the early twentieth century, having been a critical factor, particularly in Britain, in moving towards 'a highly interventionist state apparatus, within a relatively impoverished productive system'.[40] Also, by this time, the urban–rural mortality differential had diminished. In fact, in some urban systems the larger cities were significantly healthier than those places further down the hierarchy.[41] Furthermore, we have also deliberately limited our selection of papers to those which consider public health, rather than health, or medicine, or health care. However, we have been conscious of the domination of the historiography of public health by an essentially nineteenth-century 'environmentalist' agenda, and we hope that we have provided some indications of the value of a broader definition and the potential offered by some refocused conceptual tools.

---

[39]   Law, 'Growth of Urban Population'.
[40]   A. Sutcliffe, 'In Search of the Urban Variable: Britain in the Later Nineteenth Century', in A. Sutcliffe and D. Fraser (eds), *The Pursuit of Urban History* (London, 1983), p. 263.
[41]   G. Kearns, 'Zivilis or Hygaeia: urban public health and the epidemiologic transition', in R. Lawton (ed.), *The Rise and Fall of Great Cities: Aspects of Urbanisation in the Western World* (London, 1989), pp. 96–124.

2

Ritual and public health in the early medieval city

Peregrine Horden

> It would be an error to put ... [public] works in a category by themselves
> as 'utilitarian' in opposition to 'religious' works such as temples.
> Temples are just as utilitarian as dams and canals, since they are
> necessary to prosperity; dams and canals are as ritual as temples, since
> they are part of the same social system of seeking welfare. If *we* call
> reservoirs 'utilitarian' it is because *we* believe in their efficacy; *we* do not
> call temples so because *we* do not believe in their efficacy for the crops.[1]

A temple is as useful as a dam

The following discussion of ritual and public health takes the form of a sermon
with two texts. Above is the first text. It comes from *Kings and Councillors*, a
monograph, published in 1936, by that neglected pioneer of British social
anthropology, Arthur Maurice Hocart. Like Fustel de Coulanges in *The Ancient
City*, Hocart set out to trace the origins of social institutions back to archaic
ritual. Like Frazer's in *The Golden Bough*, Hocart's key ritual was one that
promoted fertility.[2] But Hocart was a greater scholar than Frazer and far more
wide-ranging than Fustel. In the quotation above, he is writing about public
works in general. So his main point applies *a fortiori* to public health projects.
And that main point, to repeat, is: 'temples are just as utilitarian as dams and
canals'.

In writing the history of health care, it is clearly important to respect
indigenous categories in the way that Hocart demands. If we also employ our
own concepts, it must be solely because they permit analytical refinements that
help us find our way around the world of the people we are investigating. My
second text illustrates how the balance can be struck, while unconsciously

---

[1]   A.M. Hocart, *Kings and Councillors: An Essay in the Comparative Anatomy of
Human Society*, first published Cairo, 1936, repr. ed. R. Needham (Chicago and London,
1970), p. 217.

[2]   On Hocart see Needham's long introduction to his edition of *Kings and Councillors*.

echoing Hocart on the significance and efficacy of ritual. In her fine book about charity in early modern Turin, Sandra Cavallo politely chides historians for interpreting plague measures of the sixteenth century simplistically in terms of the broad social and economic *conjoncture* and the workings of the centralised state. A much more local and finely-tuned approach is called for, she argues: first, to the politics of plague prevention; and second, also, to the way in which we try to evaluate the measures taken.

'The elaborate segregation and disinfection measures adopted within cities', Cavallo writes,

> undoubtedly had an important role on the *symbolic* level (based as they were on notions of physical contamination and *purification*), and on the *ritual* level (contributing for example to preserve a sense of community and to discourage anti-social behaviour). But these aspects of the question are yet to be analysed, while most studies of the plague tend instead to look at anti-plague practices from the point of view of the impact they had on the disease itself.[3]

Those are the two texts. The message of the sermon they are intended to introduce is this. In the history of pre-modern – let us say, pre-nineteenth-century – public health measures, sewers and skeletons are not quite enough. A materialist–biological account will clearly capture some of the story. It will tell us about 'public health' as the *object* of policy: public ill health, as it usually turns out. But it will do that only in the narrow terms of biomedicine and demography, ignoring other aspects of the sort that Cavallo mentions, such as purification, or the sense of community. A materialist account will also tell us about the *instruments* of policy: the measures taken to promote collective health and combat epidemics. But it will do that legalistically, in terms only of centrally-framed 'practical' regulations. And these will have been selected for consideration primarily because they conform to our secular and biomedically-inspired notions of what public health promotion involves. My contention in this chapter is that this should not be the whole story. After all, medical historians no longer think that the only question worth asking of a pre-modern drug concerns its biological efficacy. 'Did it work?' deserves – and nowadays usually evokes – a more subtle response. And yet, by contrast, two of the liveliest controversies in the historiography of modern public health have revolved entirely around material questions: I refer to the McKeown debate and the question of whether quarantine measures were the reason why the plague came to an end in Europe.[4] This materialist approach will not, I submit, enable

---

[3]   S. Cavallo, *Charity and Power in Early Modern Italy: Benefactors and their Motives in Turin, 1541–1789* (Cambridge, 1995), pp. 44–5, 47 (quotation, italics added).

[4]   On McKeown and his critics, R.M. Smith, 'Demography and Medicine', in W.F. Bynum and R. Porter (eds), *Companion Encyclopedia of the History of Medicine* (London,

us to understand why pre-modern European public health measures evolved as they did. A broader conception of the topic is called for: one that gives due weight to ritual and symbolism, as we define them; and one that, equally, takes past conceptions of health seriously and does not just Whiggishly seek out foreshadowings of what was to come in the industrial age. The symbolic may be as important as the material. That is, purity and community may be as desirable as health in a biomedical sense. A temple is as useful as a dam.

Plague and piety

Let me now try to illustrate what one chapter in a non-materialist account of public health might look like. It is in the measures to contain the spread of the Black Death in the fourteenth century that general accounts of public health often locate the first stirrings of real modernity.[5] And it is in terms of 'strategies for collective health' that such general accounts often define public health.[6] So let us stay with plague for the moment (other diseases can enter the discussion later), and let us ask what strategies for curtailing the plague epidemics of the early Middle Ages (c. 300–1000) were favoured by those in charge of cities.

There is, unfortunately, no early medieval concept under which these strategies can readily be grouped. *Salus publica*, we know, was not quite what was at stake. As an explicit aim of government, that term possessed too broad a range of essentially political and ethical meanings – focusing on the idea of 'the common good' – to be quite to the point.[7] Was there, however, an unlabelled, implicit notion of a public health measure equivalent in scope and method to those of the later Middle Ages?

> When the bubonic plague was cruelly assailing the population within the walls of the city of Trier, the priest of God [Nicetius] assiduously implored divine mercy for the sheep entrusted to him. Suddenly, in the night, a great noise was heard, like a violent clap of thunder which broke

1993), 2, pp. 1663–92. P. Slack, 'The Disappearance of Plague: An Alternative View', *Economic History Review*, 2nd series, 34 (1981), 469–76.

[5]   K. Park, 'Medicine and Society in Medieval Europe, 500–1500', in A. Wear (ed.), *Medicine in Society* (Cambridge, 1992), pp. 86–7; D. Porter, 'Public Health', in Bynum and Porter, *Companion Encyclopedia*, 2, pp. 1231–3; *eadem, Health, Civilization and the State: A History of Public Health from Ancient to Modern Times* (London and New York, 1999), p. 31; A.G. Carmichael, 'History of Public Health and Sanitation in the West before 1700', in K.F. Kiple (ed.), *The Cambridge World History of Human Disease* (Cambridge, 1993), p. 197. Cf. G. Rosen, *A History of Public Health*, first published 1958, expanded edn (Baltimore and London, 1993), pp. 41–2.

[6]   D. Porter, 'Public Health', p. 1231; compare *eadem, Health*, p. 4.

[7]   J.H. Burns (ed.), *The Cambridge History of Medieval Political Thought c. 350–c. 1450* (Cambridge, 1988), pp. 24, 143.

above the bridge over the river, so that one would have thought that the town was going to be split in two. And all the people were lying in their beds, filled with terror and hiding from the coming of death. And one could hear in the midst of the noise a voice clearer than the others, saying 'What must we do, companions? For at one of the gates Bishop Eucherius watches, and at the other Maximin is on the alert. Nicetius is busy in the middle. There is nothing left for us to do except leave the town in their protection.' As soon as this voice had been heard, the malady ceased, and from that moment no-one else died. Thus we cannot doubt that the town had been protected by the power of the bishop.[8]

The author is Gregory, Bishop of Tours, the great hagiographer of Frankish Gaul. He was writing in the 590s, from the personal information of one of Bishop Nicetius's protégés. This man became a distinguished abbot and, according to Gregory, a miracle-worker himself – with a speciality in water management.[9] Nicetius died in 564 or later. Like many bishop-saints of this early phase of the post-Roman West, he had established himself, if a little precariously, as the all-purpose public authority and administrator of his city.[10] In the words of the foremost preacher of the time, he was its 'superinspector'.[11] We cannot know what events gave rise to the miracle story that was passed to Gregory some forty years later. We can be reasonably confident that the epidemic referred to was the wave of bubonic plague which spread across Europe in 543, the year after it first reached and ravaged Constantinople.[12] But that is the limit of our information; and I do not want to speculate, on the basis of this evidence, about what anyone alive in Trier during the plague actually did or thought. It is more important, first, to look at the text itself and then, second, to ask about its presumed purpose.

One major theme in the extract is space. The scene depicted is bounded by the city's walls. The plague rages within those walls. A crisis is reached – a crisis in the strict sense of the turning point of an illness. A clap of thunder

---

[8]   Gregory of Tours, *Life of the Fathers*, 17.4, trans. E. James (Liverpool, 1985), pp. 118–19.

[9]   *Books of Histories* [*History of the Franks*], 10.29. (Primary sources that may for present purposes be consulted in any accessible edition are cited, as here, by standard subdivision of the text rather than by page.) E. Ewig, *Trier im Merowingerreich* (Trier, 1954), pp. 97ff.

[10]   P. Brown, *The Rise of Western Christendom* (Oxford and Cambridge, MA, 1996), ch. 6 for context. P. Horden, 'Disease, Dragons and Saints: The Management of Epidemics in the Dark Ages', in T. Ranger and P. Slack (eds), *Epidemics and Ideas* (Cambridge, 1992), pp. 73–4 for basic references. F. Prinz, 'Die Bischöfliche Stadtherrschaft im Frankenreich vom 5. bis zum 7. Jahrhundert', *Historische Zeitschrift*, 217 (1974), 1–35, also more for sources than for interpretation.

[11]   Caesarius of Arles, *Sermon*, 1.19.

[12]   J.-N. Biraben and J. Le Goff, 'The Plague in the Early Middle Ages', in R. Forster and O. Ranum (eds), *Biology of Man in History* (Baltimore and London, 1975), pp. 48–80 (trans. from *Annales* [November–December 1969], 1484–1510), remains fundamental.

seems to be about to bisect the city by breaking its central bridge. As we would gloss it: under the impact of the epidemic, the city is disintegrating as a social entity. The people are abed, but in a state of panic – the reverse of how dutiful citizens should behave, especially at night. It is easy to see why they are panicking, however. This epidemic is caused by demons, a purposeful, integrated group: their 'spokesman' addresses them as companions. What defeats them are the prayers of Nicetius conjoined with those of two of his predecessors. (This is not a community as sociologists have tried to define it, but one that embraces the dead as well as the living.) All three bishops are strategically placed. Between them they define the key aspects of urban space, its margins and its centre. The dead ones are suitably liminal: they are both present in their tombs in the city and yet absent, in the presence of God, with whom they intercede. They act as gatekeepers. Nicetius, as the central living authority, holds the centre. (By implication, he could even perhaps be 'keeping the bridge'.) The metaphor is, above all, military. The demons of plague lift their progressive occupation of urban space because the city's leaders are too vigilant for them ('Eucherius watches … Maximin is on the alert'). No reader of Susan Sontag needs to be reminded of how often military metaphors have 'invaded' evocations of disease both literary and scientific.[13] Analogies with the vigilant control of urban space and its boundaries by later health boards would not be entirely fanciful. I suggest that the symbolic equivalence underlying the passage is, however, that of topographical space and social coherence – assaulted, threatened with disintegration, restored.

The conception of health here is more ample than that of biomedicine. In 1946 the World Health Organization famously, and rashly, defined health as 'a state of complete physical, mental and social well-being' – a state seldom attainable outside California. 'Social well-being': it requires no great familiarity with medical anthropology, no subscription to the journal *Culture, Medicine and Psychiatry*, to realise the importance of the social dimension of health. Ill health may quite simply be equated with social dysfunction, as it is, implicitly, by many of the peoples whom anthropologists have studied; or it may be seen as the somatisation, in the individual, of tensions in the family or wider society, a model of social disorder fashioned by and upon the body.[14] Either way, health is no purely personal matter. It is interpersonal: not so much psycho- as socio-somatic.[15]

Health is also spiritual. So Gregory of Tours would have argued. To the WHO definition another dimension should be added: one that partakes of the

[13]   S. Sontag, *Aids and its Metaphors*, Penguin edn (London, 1989), pp. 9–11.

[14]   See among a vast anthropological literature, M. Herzfeld, 'Closure as Cure: Tropes in the Exploration of Bodily and Social Disorder', *Current Anthropology*, 27 (1986), 107–20.

[15]   For the relevant historical application of such notions, see R. Van Dam, *Leadership and Community in Late Antique Gaul* (Berkeley and Los Angeles, 1985), pp. 259–60.

mental and the social but goes beyond both. The health of the community that resides in its good internal relations derives ultimately from the relations between the populace and their Maker. The supreme physicians – and therefore the supreme public health promoters – are *Christus medicus*, His healing saints, and confessors as the physicians of individual souls. This is not, of course, to say that all illness was thought to stem from specific, individual sins. Different kinds of aetiology – divine, demonic, natural – might be variously invoked according to context. But the profound connection between the health of the soul and that of the body was held to be inescapable throughout the Middle Ages and, of course, beyond.[16] To the progress or prevention of a plague, the spiritual condition of its likely victims was no irrelevance.[17] In the fourteenth century a learned Spanish physician could analyse 'moral' and 'natural' pestilence side by side, placing them on an equal ontological footing. Until the mid-Victorian age, the English epithet 'pestilent' could mean 'injurious ... to religion, morals, or public peace'.[18]

The remedies for pestilence extended, then, beyond solidarity to collective prayer and penitence. Such I take to be the message of Gregory's little narration quoted above: its intended effects on thought and action. Support your bishop; accept his place in the line of worthies; trust in divine mercy; and above all make yourselves worthy of that mercy. That is what he wants to convey. That is the best prophylactic, the best 'collective strategy' to avert future returns of the epidemic, the way to dispel the demons of a disorder that is at once physical (plague), social (disintegration) and spiritual (sin). A temple is as practical as a dam – and a miracle is as practical as a health board.

Other texts from Gregory's corpus of hagiographies make clear the connection between the demonstration of saintly episcopal power and collective responses to plague. When the same epidemic was threatening Rheims, Gregory reports, the people rushed to the tomb of their dead patron saint, Remigius.[19] They kept vigil, singing hymns and psalms.

> At dawn they searched in a treatise for what was still missing from their request [for protection]. By the revelation of God they discovered how,

---

[16]   J. Agrimi and C. Crisciani, 'Medicina del corpo e medicina dell'anima: note sul sapere del medico fino all'inizio del sec. XIII', *Episteme*, 10 (1976), 5–102; C. Rawcliffe, 'Medicine for the Soul: the Medieval English Hospital and the Quest for Spiritual Health', in J.R. Hinnells and R. Porter (eds) *Religion, Health and Suffering* (London and New York, 1999), pp. 316–38.

[17]   See R. Horrox, *The Black Death* (Manchester and New York, 1994), ch. 3, esp. pp. 97–8 for fourteenth-century parallels.

[18]   J. Arrizabalaga, 'Facing the Black Death: Perceptions and Reactions of University Medical Practitioners', in L. García-Ballester et al. (eds), *Practical Medicine from Salerno to the Black Death* (Cambridge, 1994), pp. 244–5; *OED*, 2nd edn, 'pestilent' 3, with Sontag, *Illness as Metaphor*, Penguin edn (Harmondsworth, 1983), p. 63.

[19]   Gregory, *Glory of the Confessors*, 78, trans. R. Van Dam (Liverpool, 1988), pp. 82–3. See also *Books of Histories*, 9.22.

after first praying, they might fortify the defenses of the city with a still more effective defense.

What was missing from their previous efforts was a (symbolic) appropriation of urban space. They took the saint's funeral shroud and arranged it in the shape of a bier. Carrying crosses and candles, they processed the shroud around the city and also around its suburban villages and any outlying solitary dwellings. Plague approached the edge of the city.

> It advanced all the way to the spot where the relic of the blessed Remigius had gone, and whenever it recognized the boundary that had been set, it did not in any way dare to advance further.

The disease even relinquished places it had previously invaded. There was thus containment as well as prevention – reordering of space, a separation of the sacred and the diseased.

Such collective responses do not merely belong in the literary realm of hagiography. They could rapidly be institutionalised. When plague ravaged the region of Arles, Gallus Bishop of Clermont, Gregory's uncle, interceded for his people. He was, Gregory tells us, assured by an angel that his prayer had been heard and that, while he was alive, no one would succumb to the disease. So, Gregory continues, 'he instituted the prayers called Rogations'.[20] Actually, Gallus seems to have made a special Lenten addition to the cycle of penitential processions that had developed since the fourth century. What had begun as a collective prayer for good harvest – shades of Hocart – could be additionally pressed into service as a remedy for public health hazards and other disasters. Along the Persian Gulf, the Rogation processions of Nestorian bishops had cleared the waters of giant sharks, to the benefit of the local pearl fishers.[21] Plague control was, though, their main health-related purpose in the sixth-century West. In Rome in 590, shortly before Gregory set down the first of the vignettes quoted above, Pope Gregory the Great exhorted the population of the stricken city to contrition. He then divided them up by religious calling – priests, monks, laity and so on – and had each group process from a different church to converge at S. Maria Maggiore. A ritual of penitence and social cohesion combined – not to be thought the less utilitarian or efficacious for the fact that some eighty people reportedly fell dead of plague during the great assembly.[22] Rogations, to follow the verdict of Michael Wallace-Hadrill, 'demonstrated in a dramatic way how the Church could identify local disaster with local sin and provide the remedy in a communal act of propitiation that

---

[20]   *Life of the Fathers*, 6.6 (pp. 57–8).
[21]   Brown, *Rise of Western Christendom*, p. 173.
[22]   Gregory of Tours, *Books of Histories*, 10.1; cf. 9.20.

involved everyone' – not least, it should be added, the rich, who might otherwise have added to the social dislocation by running off (in the words of a preacher, like deserters from an army).[23] Those who shunned the remedy of repentance reportedly found their houses marked with the Greek letter T, or perhaps a cross. Gregory, who provides the report, knew this well from his own family tradition.[24]

So far I have been looking at plague, and at what (following Cavallo) we might label ritual and symbolism in plague control. I have been concentrating on what some might be tempted to think of as a merely religious approach to containing an epidemic. Of course, it is a commonplace of the historiography of plague in later centuries that folk aetiologies, whether learned or lay, had God as the author of pestilence and contrition as its best remedy[25] (even if the connection between the soul's and the body's health was sometimes learnedly 'medicalised' in terms of one of the 'non-naturals').[26] I am arguing, however, for a slightly different approach to religious responses.

First (Hocart's point about practicality) they have to be treated as part of 'the real thing'. They are not a curious by-way from the main subject of public health. Granted, much of the early medieval evidence for them is literary: hagiographical vignettes. Yet literary representations – it hardly needs stating in these 'post-postmodern' days – have their own interest, value and potency. And at the time of their first hearing, they were widely held to represent genuine events. Moreover, these events were not from some age of miracles in a golden past, but, in Gregory's own case, sometimes quite recent 'family affairs'. Nor did the texts just celebrate past achievements. They furnished the attentive with models for both collective and individual action in averting future epidemics.

Second, the collective aspect needs to be given more emphasis than is usually the case with plague historians' glancing references to processions. The ritual procedures reviewed above were (ideally) corporate strategies for collective health that operated in a complex way, under a suitably broad definition of well-being. What they demonstrate is not miraculous power operating in, as it were, a blinding flash but, rather, certain *techniques* for the reconfiguration of urban space. And these techniques are often shown being deployed at the instigation of a particular style of urban leadership – one which in vigour and comprehensiveness bears comparison with that of any Renaissance health board.

---

[23]   J.M. Wallace-Hadrill, *The Frankish Church* (Oxford, 1983), p. 11. Brown, *Rise of Western Christendom*, p. 63. Caesarius, *Sermon* 133.
[24]   *Glory of the Martyrs*, 50, trans. Van Dam (Liverpool, 1988), 76; *Books of Histories*, 4.5.
[25]   For example Horrox, *Black Death*.
[26]   Arrizabalaga, 'Facing the Black Death', p. 280.

Finally, since historians tend to associate religious responses to public health with periods of crisis, it should be added that none of the foregoing arguments relates exclusively to plague epidemics. Other less threatening diseases were supposed to have been effaced by dramatic gestures made at the centre of things. Gregory's was a time in which the conversion of the Western barbarians to Catholic Christianity was recent and patchy. So he illustrates the potential effect of conversion on the collective health of a whole population. The leprosy of heresy was no mere metaphor.[27] When the King of the Suevi (in Galicia) and his household accepted Catholic baptism,

> the people were freed from loathsome leprosy, and all ill people were cured; to the present day the disease of leprosy has never appeared on anyone there.[28]

As for still less threatening, characteristically endemic disease, I have suggested elsewhere that bishops who are figured in hagiography as taming dragons should perhaps be understood as symbolically facing up to the challenge of malaria.[29]

Sacraments and pollutions

All such spectacular and literally space-saving 'miracles of public health' (as I dare to call them) were, in many respects, simply occasional magnifications of commonplace rituals that, in the Christian urban communities of the early medieval West, were meant to involve everyone and to promote collective well-being. I shall pass them rapidly in review before focusing on what may have been a still more basic level of 'public health' activity by the church: countering pollution.

There were festivals of saints and martyrs – 'rituals of consensus', social healing, as processions were also intended to be.[30] Preparation to join in such festivals could involve an examination of conscience that had strong implications for somatic health. 'Woe is me,' reportedly lamented a blind

---

[27]   See R.I. Moore, 'Heresy as Disease', in D.W. Lourdaux and D. Verhelst (eds), *The Concept of Heresy in the Middle Ages* (Louvain, 1976), pp. 1–11.

[28]   *Virtuti Martini*, 1.11, trans. Van Dam, *Saints and their Miracles in Late Antique Gaul* (Princeton, 1993), p. 213.

[29]   'Disease, Dragons and Saints'. See now also P. Squatriti, 'Water, Nature and Culture in Early Medieval Lucca', *Early Medieval Europe*, 4 (1995), 21–40, similarly drawing a connection between hagiography and environmental management.

[30]   P. Brown, *The Cult of the Saints* (London, 1981), pp. 99–100. See also W.E. Klingshirn, *Caesarius of Arles: The Making of a Christian Community in Late Antique Gaul* (Cambridge, 1994), ch. 7.

woman unable to participate on such an occasion, 'who does not deserve to see this festival with the rest of the congregation, because I have been blinded by my sins!'[31] Prayer restored her sight and enabled her to set off for church. At the festivals themselves, possessions were not simply publicised but perhaps actually induced, and exorcisms were achieved, as the troubled worked through whatever dysfunctions were being somatised into demons within.[32]

More common than great miracles and repeated festivals were the sacraments. Indeed, to the question of what preventive public health measures would have been seen by the élites of Gregory's time as the truly essential, the most far-reaching, one tempting answer would be: baptism and the Eucharist. In these, individual and collective responsibilities merged. Baptism was the equivalent of childhood inoculation: the means to forgiveness of original sin and an exorcism, a rebirth into health.[33] The Eucharist, for both the congregation of observers and the smaller number of actual communicants, was, like the saint's festival which periodically framed it, a ritual of social integration.[34] Presence at it could bring obviously beneficial results: Gregory's mother had saved their household from plague by attending mass.[35]

The last sacrament to be mentioned in this brief review is penance. Gregory's was a time when an ancient system of public one-off penance for very serious sins was just beginning to give way to a private, repeatable, more nuanced transaction between confessor and penitent – a transaction concerning venial sins. The sins might be punished by minor (though not trivial) penances, according to a tariff set out in a penitential. Penitentials are first evident in Ireland but were soon exported to Britain and the Continent. As a body of texts, they bear witness to an attempt by early medieval churches to regulate a significant number of the daily thoughts and activities of priests themselves, as well as of monks and other laity.[36] Penitentials deal with Catholic devotion, paganism and magic; also with the deadly sins, not least those of the stomach and the loins. No systematic or evenly-distributed system of control was ever possible or envisaged. None the less this material does manifest, if only partially and indirectly, what can be seen as corporate priestly concerns for communal health – health under a variety of descriptions. The common way of

---

[31]   *Virtuti Martini*, 2.28, trans. Van Dam, 243.
[32]   Compare Brown, *Cult of the Saints*, p. 111.
[33]   A. Angenendt, 'Der Taufritus im frühen Mittelalter', *Settimane Spoleto*, 33 (1985), 275–321; H.A. Kelly, *The Devil at Baptism* (Ithaca, 1985); P. Cramer, *Baptism and Change in the Early Middle Ages c. 200–c. 1150* (Cambridge, 1993), pp. 136ff.
[34]   Van Dam, *Saints and their Miracles*, p. 93; Klingshirn, *Caesarius*, pp. 155–8.
[35]   *Glory of the Martyrs*, 50, trans. Van Dam, 76; *Books of Histories*, 4.5.
[36]   Brown, *Rise of Western Christendom*, pp. 158–61. A.J. Frantzen, *The Literature of Penance in Anglo-Saxon England* (New Brunswick, 1983).

characterising penitentials as setting out 'health-giving medicine for souls' was, like the leprosy of heresy, far from metaphoric.[37]

On a modern definition of health, the dietary prescriptions that are dotted around the penitential corpus have been seen as promoting hygiene in food preparation. ('If anyone accidentally touches food with unwashed hands ...', as one canon begins.)[38] Other canons which attempt to promote moderation and propriety in matters of alcohol as well as food, in sex and the expression of anger, could be seen as encouraging bodily health, as well as helping reduce that sinfulness which is the harbinger of epidemics. But that is not the reason why penitentials should be important to historians of early medieval public health. Their significance is that they remind us again of the need to relativise the measures we are considering – relativise them to local conceptions of health and well-being. On the question of diet, for instance, what is evident in these sources is not hygiene but 'ethno-hygiene', and of a perhaps unsettling kind. After all, the canon just quoted about touching food with unwashed hands excuses the omission if it was unintentional – just as it goes on to excuse allowing a mouse to touch the food. Such dietary and seemingly hygienic prescriptions can no more be accounted for in modern biological or medical terms than can those of Leviticus. Rather than hygiene, these penitentials aim to promote purity and the avoidance of pollution. Their enemy is not so much dirt as uncleanness.

Now this is not the usual stuff of public health historiography. Narratives conventionally concentrate on those areas in which a pre-modern conception of miasma or corrupt air coincides quite neatly with our contemporary notions of the sources of environmental pollution: sullied water, human and animal waste, and so on. Yet a broader or perhaps different conception of pollution is evoked by these penitential texts: certainly an elusive one. Despite the best efforts of philologists and anthropologists, it remains an 'umbrella' term. We feebly differentiate it from its material equivalent by labelling it 'ritual pollution'; an unsatisfactory solution, because the ritual aspect often seems to subsume the material.[39] For all its ambiguity the term 'pollution' does, however, adequately

[37] *Penitential of Cummean*, prologue, trans. J.T. McNeill and H.M. Gamer, *Medieval Handbooks of Penance*, first published 1938 (repr. New York, 1965), p. 99. For details of editions and further references supporting much of what follows see R. Meens, 'Pollution in the Early Middle Ages: The Case of the Food Regulations in Penitentials', *Early Medieval Europe*, 4 (1995), 3–19. Also *idem*, 'The Frequency and Nature of Early Medieval Penance', in P. Biller and A.J. Minnis (eds), *Handling Sin: Confession in the Middle Ages* (York, 1998), pp. 35–61.

[38] *Penitential of Theodore*, 7.7 (McNeill and Gamer, p. 191).

[39] M. Douglas, *Purity and Danger: An Analysis of the Concepts of Pollution and Taboo* (London, 1966), enjoys a higher reputation among historians than among anthropologists. See further R. Parker, *Miasma: Pollution and Purification in Early Greek Religion* (Oxford, 1983); A.S. Meigs, 'A Papuan Perspective on Pollution', *Man*, n.s. 13 (1978), 304–18; Meens, 'Pollution'.

reflect the vocabulary of the Latin texts.[40] It refers to a cluster of acts or states which are characteristically dangerous – and often contagious too. And these acts and states (we can generalise) have the property of being fully intelligible as pollutants only in religious and cosmological terms, even when they are described in a quasi-medical way.

As a further illustration: members of some of the congregations in which the penitentials were applied seem to have regarded the consumption of urine and excrement, scabs, lice, blood and semen as beneficial to health.[41] But in punishing such beliefs – which are by no means without their analogues in other periods and places – the confessors were far from combating superstition with hygienic rationalism.[42] Rather, they were trying to replace one set of pollution ideas with another. A canon in an Anglo-Saxon penitential states: 'the hare may be eaten, and it is good for dysentery; and its gall is to be mixed with pepper for [the relief of] pain'.[43] The medical advantage is paraded, but the ulterior motive is to encourage the view that the hare – despite Leviticus 11.6 – is a 'clean' animal. In similar spirit, the next canon in the same collection allows the consumption of the honey of homicidal bees (although the bees themselves should be killed). Pollution is contagious but not that contagious, or at least not in that particular fashion.[44] On the other hand, the meat of the offspring of an animal that has been party to bestiality should be strenuously avoided. In that case the pollution, a Lamarckian inheritance, remains powerful. Again, by way of final example, to drink the 'leavings' of a dog is obviously dirty, polluting – but no more or less so than to drink those of a thief or a man guilty of incest.[45]

So far I have stressed 'ritual pollution' for two main reasons. First, the concept gives us a view of public health from the receiving end – a view that avoids anachronistic 'biologism'. It shows ritual as being crucial to an understanding of public health *objectives*, as well as measures. Second, it introduces the church at work in a decentralised, indeed uncoordinated manner, promoting 'socio-somatic' well-being. And this, I submit, constitutes a level of activity beneath (or beyond) the church's other sacramental interventions in collective ill-health, as well as those more dramatic miracles wrought by virtuoso bishops with which I began. But pollution can be a useful heading in other ways, too. Its history hints at still further levels of activity – harder to document, scarcely institutionalised, but equally relevant to an assessment of

---

[40]   Meens, 'Pollution', p. 23.
[41]   Ibid., pp. 12–13.
[42]   H. von Staden, 'Women and Dirt', *Helios*, 19 (1992), 7–30 (classical); Parker, *Miasma*, pp. 231, 233–4 (late antique).
[43]   *Penitential of Theodore*, 11.5 (p. 208).
[44]   Meens, 'Pollution', pp. 6, 12–13.
[45]   *Old Irish Penitential*, 17 (p. 159).

urban health and of means of enhancing it in the early Middle Ages. Moreover the concept will, later, provide a way of bringing material considerations back into the picture without distorting their early medieval significance.[46]

Let us explore that sub-institutional level a little further. The theme common to the different types of activity that I have tried to identify is the demarcation and management of space in the city: topographical space, as in those miracles; social space in church festivals; ritual space (for want of a more sensitive term) in the penitentials, involving the separation of the clean from the unclean, the sacred from the polluted. I suggest that church leaders might be thought of as attempting, through subtle adjustments as much as through grand gestures or regulations, to harmonise topographical and ritual space.

They can be seen to do so in three ways: firstly, in the charitable foundations and outdoor relief services that they established or administered for the benefit of the very poor.[47] Of course, the nursing and sustenance provided might have been just sufficient in aggregate to affect the overall health of the urban population – health defined in its modern sense. But the activities in question should also, perhaps, be seen in terms of the management of pollution. At least some of the poor were, I hypothesise, seen as polluted and contagious because of their immorality, their contacts with criminals and animals, the unclean food upon which they, of necessity, sometimes depended,[48] and their diseases (not least leprosy, towards which attitudes could be as hard in this period as in the thirteenth century).[49] They needed purification or, where that was impossible, a certain amount of segregation – not in a draconian anticipation of *renfermement*, but through the allocation of particular urban spaces, in shrines, hospitals, bishops' houses and the like.[50]

Beliefs in the pollution of death, secondly, had to be managed in a different way. To summarise crudely a lengthy and complex process, we could say that the Church turned the topography inherited from the ancient city, not only inside out but also, more pertinently in this context, *outside* in. On one influential argument, it turned the city inside out through the emphasis it gave

---

[46] On the dangers of 'medical materialism' in interpreting pollution beliefs, Douglas, *Purity and Danger*, pp. 29–32, Parker, *Miasma*, pp. 57–8, and Meens, 'Pollution', p. 5, are salutary.

[47] See for example T. Sternberg, *Orientalium More Secutus: Räume und Institutionen der Caritas des 5. bis 7. Jahrhunderts in Gallien* (Münster, 1991).

[48] P. Bonnassie, 'Consommation d'aliments immondes et cannibalisme de survie dans l'Occident du Haut Moyen Age', *Annales* (September–October 1989), 1035–56.

[49] The extreme instance, not yet adequately explained, is the Lombard Edict of Rothar, cap. 176.

[50] For comparison with the central Middle Ages see R. Gilchrist, 'Christian Bodies and Souls: The Archaeology of Life and Death in Later Medieval Hospitals', in S. Bassett (ed.), *Death in Towns: Urban Responses to the Dying and the Dead 100–1600* (Leicester, 1992), pp. 112–15.

to religious festivals associated with suburban or peripheral shrines.[51] It turned the city outside in through the admission of intramural burials – burials in the space that ancient society had studiously kept free of their pollution. On this front, it was not the contagion itself that had to be countered but beliefs about its source.[52]

With the third kind of pollution that belongs in this context, the task was the converse. Recognition of a new kind of defilement had to be encouraged: that of an only recently and unevenly suppressed paganism. Demons now embodied the uncleanness lurking in the remains of the cult sites of the old religion. New rules of avoidance and containment were needed if possession was not to become epidemic. Congregations had to be taught how to negotiate a fresh and highly threatening demonic geography.[53]

The case for materialism

In the foregoing, it will seem as if I have done little more than endorse George Rosen's brief account of my topic in his history of public health.

> In the West during the earlier medieval period ... health problems were for the most part considered and dealt with in magical and religious terms ... prayer, penitence and the invocation of saints were the means employed to deal with health problems ... Whatever knowledge concerning health and hygiene survived was ... applied in the hygienic arrangements and regulations of the monastic communities.[54]

Rosen was writing in the 1950s, under the entirely pardonable influence of what now seems like a Dark-Age view of the Dark Ages, as sunk irremediably in superstition and seriously deficient in rational medicine. Of course, early medieval medicine nowadays receives a fuller and more understanding press.[55] And I hope to have shown that religious approaches to public health should be treated with equal sympathy. There are, however, two more substantial points to register in protest at a pessimistic view of the period which, under this

---

[51]   Brown, *Cult of the Saints*, pp. 4–8.

[52]   J. Harries, 'Death and the Dead in the Late Roman West', in Bassett, *Death in Towns*, pp. 57–9.

[53]   Brown, *Cult of the Saints*, p. 125; Klingshirn, *Caesarius of Arles*, ch. 6. For the notion of a demonic geography see references in Horden, 'Responses to Possession and Insanity in the Earlier Byzantine World', *Social History of Medicine*, 6 (1993), 182–3.

[54]   Rosen, *History of Public Health*, pp. 28–9.

[55]   See M.L. Cameron, *Anglo-Saxon Medicine* (Cambridge, 1993), for an extreme defence of the rationality of 'Dark-Age' therapeutics. Contrast F. Wallis, 'The Experience of the Book: Manuscripts, Texts and the Role of Epistemology in Early Medieval Medicine', in D. Bates (ed.), *Knowledge and the Scholarly Medical Traditions* (Cambridge, 1995), pp. 101–26.

heading of public health, survives essentially unaltered in more recent accounts.[56]

First, even on the materialist definition of what constitutes the history of public health, the early Middle Ages were not the dispiriting blank they are still often taken to have been. That is, between the glories of the Roman aqueduct and the environmental regulations of the thirteenth-century Italian communes (regulations that have plausibly been connected to the revival of Roman law) something *did* happen. Monasteries were no more the only centres of hygiene than they were the only guardians of classical culture. There is another article to be written on public health measures that would be the obverse of this one. It could place ritual and symbolism in the background and concentrate, as I have not done, on more familiar tasks: the management of drainage, water supply, perhaps even sewerage, and the oversight of food supply, as well as the provision of nursing services already mentioned.[57] It would also give some space to plague control measures – measures of a sort that would not have been out of place in the later Middle Ages, and that involved an attempt to check the spread of an epidemic by prohibiting movement between fairs.[58] Once again, the primary responsibility for all such measures lay with bishops. To revert to my opening example: besides miraculously warding off plague, Nicetius of Trier was active in poor relief, a pioneering viticulturalist, and above all a great builder – not only of churches but of a castle, its water led by conduits which also turned a mill.[59] Not exactly public health, but enterprises not very far removed from it in terms of techniques and resources. In the following century, the seventh, Desiderius of Cahors was one bishop known to have been asked to set up checkpoints to stop pestiferous merchants (presumably thought to be carrying the disease in their personal miasma). He also wrote to Gallus of Clermont, a successor to that Gallus mentioned above, asking for the loan of specialist craftsmen who could make the wooden tubing necessary for his city's refurbished water supply.[60] Correspondence about such matters seldom comes down to us from this period. It survives only when its presumed literary merits earn it a place in a 'published' letter collection. So it is reasonable to envisage such activity as having been much more frequent than its surviving attestations.

---

[56]   Carmichael, 'History of Public Health', p. 193, still privileging clean monasteries. See also Porter, *Health*, pp. 22–3 on the early Middle Ages, discussing only hospitals.

[57]   Add to references in n. 10 above: B. Ward-Perkins, *From Classical Antiquity to the Middle Ages: Urban Public Building in Northern and Central Italy* (Oxford, 1984), ch. 7 (water and water supply), esp. e.g. p. 134, sewers and drainage in early medieval Pavia. Compare Squatriti, *Water and Society in Early Medieval Italy, AD 400–1000* (Cambridge, 1998), ch. 2.

[58]   J. Durliat, 'Les attributions civiles des évêques mérovingiens: l'exemple de Didier, évêque de Cahors (630–655)', *Annales du Midi*, 91 (1979), 238–9, 244.

[59]   Venantius Fortunatus, *Carmina*, 3.11–12.

[60]   Durliat, 'Attributions', pp. 242–4.

Did the material activity somehow give rise to the hagiographical miracles? Do the miracles symbolically condense a range of more mundane performances? There may be other ways of putting it. Perhaps if we could draw up a balance sheet of all the relevant connections between 'literature' and 'life', then the net influence might have been exerted in an unexpected direction. That is, the conceptual world of the early medieval hagiography might have been the model for, and stimulus to, the practicalities. A similar possibility has, after all, been entertained by students of anti-plague strategies of the *later* Middle Ages. European readiness to seek a cause, and thus a remedy, for epidemics has been attributed to the connection widely made between illness and sin. And it has been contrasted with the predominant Muslim view of plague as 'a martyrdom and a mercy', a view much less likely to engender public health measures.[61] The problem with this particular theological interpretation of the European response to the Black Death is that positing a link between sin and epidemic was hardly an invention of Europeans in the later Middle Ages. It can be found as far back as pre-classical antiquity and so cannot be used to explain particular fourteenth-century developments.[62] It is not wholly absent from Islamic interpretations of plague.[63] Nor, finally, are public health concerns of a materialist kind alien to the Muslim tradition.[64] But those are 'local difficulties': they do not invalidate the argument's general character, which is to give religious culture an important role in the explanation of medical history.

In this context, whatever causal connections we posit, during the early Middle Ages the miraculous and the mundane, the ritual and the practical, the theological and the material are best seen as lying on a continuum – as blended ingredients in the 'medical pluralism' of public health.[65] They are no more easily separable as categories than are ritual pollution and biomedical dirt. The church had to deal with miasma in whatever form it took, whether from a pagan sanctuary or a stagnant pool, an unclean animal or a blocked drain. Here is a description of how its bishops might have operated:

---

[61]   Slack and Ranger, *Epidemics and Ideas*, p. 17, with ch. 4 (Lawrence Conrad). Cf. R. Palmer, 'The Church, Leprosy and Plague in Medieval and Early Modern Europe', *Studies in Church History*, 19 (1982), 94ff; M.W. Dols, 'The Comparative Communal Responses to the Black Death in Muslim and Christian Societies', *Viator*, 5 (1974), 275ff.

[62]   Parker, *Miasma*, p. 236.

[63]   M. Dols, *The Black Death in the Middle East* (Princeton, 1977), pp. 114–15.

[64]   L.I. Conrad, 'The Plague in the Early Medieval Near East' (unpublished PhD thesis, Princeton 1981), 392ff; *idem*, 'Die Pest und ihr soziales Umfeld im Nahen Osten des frühen Mittelalters', *Der Islam*, 73 (1996), 85–9, with references; S. Hamarneh, 'Origins and Functions of the *Hisbah* System in Islam and its Impact on the Health Professions', *Sudhoffs Archiv*, 48 (1964), 157–73.

[65]   See Slack, 'Introduction', in Slack and Ranger, *Epidemics and Ideas*, p. 11, for parallels with Far Eastern history.

Authority for the control of health was in the hands of a set of leaders which included chiefs, healers and local patriarchs. These controlled the conditions of health in several different ways. First, they were responsible for controlling the kinds of deviance which were thought to threaten communal health ... Diviners identified witches, and chiefs eliminated them ... Patriarchs ... drove out or killed polluted individuals whose presence threatened the survival of local kinship groups. These included twins, and also people with smallpox who were sent out of the village into isolation ... The same triad of healing specialists, chiefs and patriarchs regulated the use of irrigation channels, burial of the dead ... and the location of sites for human waste ... Those with authority also organized rites for communal well-being, to prevent famine, epidemics and damaging wars.[66]

The setting is Tanzania towards the end of the nineteenth century. Here, again, is a mixture of the ritual and the practical, the material and the symbolic. *Mutatis mutandis*, it describes exactly the sort of context I envisage for the hagiographies previously cited.

Autres temps

My second point in defence of the 'ritualist' approach to the history of public health is that its scope is, or ought to be, much wider than the early Middle Ages. Now historians of religion generally, it hardly needs stating, have never failed to notice that numerous deities, saints, seers or other figures (such as the scapegoat) have been seen as instrumental in protecting the health of the city, either by averting disease or by dispelling it when it has arrived, through miracle, sacrifice or purification. Nor have such historians ignored the ways in which city populations have variously found a 'strategy for collective health' in seeking to appease their divinities through invocations or processions.[67] What is lacking, I think, is a general willingness to integrate such topics from the history of religion more fully into that of public health as it is usually

---

[66]   S. Feierman, quoted in Ranger and Slack, *Epidemics and Ideas*, pp. 247–8. See also S. Feierman, 'Struggles for Control: The Social Roots of Health and Healing in Modern Africa', *African Studies Review*, 28 (1985), 117–18; G. Waite, 'Public Health in Pre-Colonial East-Central Africa', in S. Feierman and J.M. Janzen (eds), *The Social Basis of Health and Healing in Africa* (Berkeley, Los Angles and Oxford, 1992), pp. 212–31, on rainmaking and sorcery control.

[67]   See from among a vast potential bibliography, Parker, *Miasma*, pp. 7–8. E. Kearns, 'Saving the City', in O. Murray and S. Price (eds), *The Greek City* (Oxford, 1990), pp. 323–44, esp. pp. 335–6 on the scapegoat; Palmer, 'The Church, Leprosy and Plague'; P. Burke, *The Historical Anthropology of Early Modern Italy* (Cambridge, 1987), pp. 210–11.

conceived. The example set by some early modernists has not been widely followed.[68]

The last part of this chapter, therefore, strays chronologically outside the early Middle Ages to offer some partial indication of how we might proceed. The theme remains the intersection of 'material' and 'ritual' conceptions of public health, especially as they bear on the perception or management of urban space.

One obvious body of evidence to investigate is biblical and Talmudic. Indeed, this argument against medical materialism would have been easier to frame if its examples had been drawn from Jewish history. So many Jewish communities, from biblical times onward, seem to have adopted centrally directed and enforced collective 'health' policies. These included not only well-known preventive measures such as ritual hygiene, dietary observance, and the proper disposal of the dead, all of them the legal responsibility of every individual – and all of them measures which have stoutly resisted materialist interpretation. The policies also embraced a subtle range of responses to pestilence.[69] According to the Book of Numbers (16.46–8), for example, during the epidemic that followed the rebellion of Korah, Aaron (at Moses' command) took fire from the altar onto his censer and added incense, as an atonement. He then ran into the middle of the congregation. In a manner that resonates with the hagiography cited above, he stood as a symbolic barrier between the living and the dead (meaning, perhaps, the healthy and the infected). The plague was stayed. In the Mishnah and Talmud – to draw a simplified composite picture – an epidemic was defined in a precise and sophisticated manner in terms of a certain mortality rate. Its presence was to be reported to the sages, 'community leaders'. The shofar was to be blown, to warn the population but also, perhaps, to call upon the Lord for help. A public fast was to be ordained. Non-religious responses were also permissible, flight among them.

Rather than pursue the better-known rabbinic material, let me take one instance of what might be seen as a preventive health measure that has been brought to light only relatively recently, from the fringes of the ancient Jewish world. The text in question comes from the Dead Sea Scrolls famously deposited by that ascetic Jewish sect widely (though not uncontroversially)

---

[68]   For example, numerous works by Carlo Cipolla; Palmer and Burke as in previous note.

[69]   What follows is based on the classic, J. Preuss, *Biblical and Talmudic Medicine*, first published 1911, trans. F. Rosner (repr. Northvale, NJ, and London, 1993); J. Neusner, *A History of the Mishnaic Law of Purities* (Leiden, 1974–77); and N. Zilber and S. Kottek, 'Pestilence in Bible and Talmud: Some Aspects related to Public Health', *Koroth*, 9 (1985), 249–61, and 151–3. For *Numbers*, see M. Douglas, *The Doctrine of Defilement in the Book of Numbers*, Journal for the Study of the Old Testament Supplement Series 158 (Sheffield, 1993), ch. 7. For the key medieval figure see F. Rosner, 'Moses Maimonides and Preventive Medicine', *Journal of the History of Medicine and Allied Sciences*, 51 (1996), 318.

identified with the Essenes. One discourse has been deciphered about the necessity of destroying a house in which mildew has appeared. It was written in code, which is hardly to be expected of a public health measure. But the provisional specialist hypothesis is that texts of this kind were early drafts of fundamental teachings, prepared for the *Maskil* or Guardian of the community as a preliminary to being fully authorised as doctrine. Medical materialists have already picked up the scent, identifying the mildew with the potentially lethal contaminant *Stachybotrys atra*, and interpreting that in turn as the cause of the Tenth Plague of Egypt. It remains to be seen whether the explanation lies here or – more likely given the discourse's apparent descent from Leviticus (14.34–53) – in the realm of religious history.[70]

My next examples are Roman, and that might seem otiose. For the major cities of the empire, Rome itself especially, are given an honourable place in all outline histories of pre-modern public health, for their aqueducts, baths, lavatories and sewers.[71] On a crude biological scale it is, of course, easy to cut such achievements down to size. Rome, it turns out, was no more or less hygienic and healthy than any other pre-industrial metropolis.[72] And no one has demonstrated this better than Alex Scobie. But, in the present 'non-biological' context, what deserves most emphasis in his rightly influential paper is the following comment:

> There was no legal obligation for a homeowner to connect his dwelling to a public street sewer ... Extant Roman law is silent on the question of where domestic latrines were to be situated and how they were to be constructed. *The Romans were legally more concerned about the intramural burial of the dead than they were about the disposal of human and animal wastes within the city.*[73]

The relevant point is not that the much-vaunted public sewers had only a limited effect on the population as a whole. (If connected to too many dwellings the sewers would stink and might back up; and in any case human manure was too valuable to be flushed away.) The point is rather that, in the

---

[70]   S.J. Pfann, paper read to 1997 Jerusalem Qumran conference; *New York Times*, 27 July and 1 August 1997.

[71]   See also J. Scarborough, 'Roman Medicine and Public Health', in T. Ogawa (ed.), *Public Health* (Tokyo, 1981), pp. 33–74. A.T. Hodge, *Roman Aqueducts and Water Supply* (London, 1992). Cf. E.J. Gowers, 'The Anatomy of Rome from Capitol to Cloaca', *Journal of Roman Studies*, 85 (1995), 23–32.

[72]   For demographic analysis see B.D. Shaw, 'Seasons of Death: Aspects of Mortality in Imperial Rome', *Journal of Roman Studies*, 86 (1996), 100–138.

[73]   A. Scobie, 'Slums, Sanitation and Mortality in the Roman World', *Klio*, 68 (1986), 399–433, at 409, my italics. See, however, R. Laurence, 'Writing the Roman Metropolis', in H.M. Parkins (ed.), *Roman Urbanism: Beyond the Consumer City* (London, 1997), pp. 11–14, for some criticism of Scobie's method and his anachronistic standards of hygiene.

eyes of the legislators, the 'ritual' pollution of the dead – the human waste in the form of corpses given intramural burial – was of greater moment than the material pollution of the living: human waste in the form of excrement. Excrement could after all be medicinal as well as good for agriculture; bodies were dangerous, and remained so until the empire had been Christianised.

Analogous points can be made about that other focus of Rome's presumed achievement in public hygiene, the baths. Among the deities most frequently represented in the statuary of ancient *thermae* were Asclepius and Hygieia. And baths were, indeed, seen as salubrious. That is why the sick came to them, probably in considerable numbers.[74] The Emperor Hadrian reportedly ordered that the sick alone should use the baths before the eighth hour, ostensibly to separate them from the healthy.[75] But he did not, it seems, prohibit the sick from also bathing *after* the eighth hour and thus mixing with the healthy; and before this measure, if it was ever actually taken, both had presumably used the baths simultaneously. The physician Celsus advised resort to the public baths for the cure of a range of ailments, including worms, dysentery, gonorrhoea, psoriasis and bowel troubles. When it came to infected wounds, though, he counselled caution. One should avoid treating these in the baths – out of concern not for other bathers, but for the patient. The bath water, Celsus says, renders a wound dirty.[76]

Such was Roman ethno-hygiene. On materialist criteria, the Romans cannot be rated very highly. Once again, a far greater danger than biological infection was perceived, a danger of an immaterial kind. The bath could be the setting of magical practices – curses and love charms alike might be thrown into the water. The bath was also the haunt of the souls of the dead and of demons.[77] The apocryphal Acts of John includes the story of a demon that religiously (as one might say) strangled a young bather of either sex three times a year. Similar stories of demons who torture or kill bathers are to be found in the hagiography of Gregory of Tours: Christianised versions of a very ancient theme.

Like human waste, then, baths belong as much to the topography of ritual pollution and supernatural danger as they do to that of somatic health. And it was the former topography that preoccupied the elites of ancient cities. The aedile, the foremost of several Roman officials some of whose functions loosely corresponded to those of modern public health inspectors, was more concerned with the city's morals than with its drains.

---

[74]   Scobie, 'Slums', 425.
[75]   *Historia Augusta*, Life of Hadrian, 22.7.
[76]   Celsus, *de Medicina*, 5.26.28C.
[77]   For references supporting what follows, K.M.D. Dunbabin, '*Baiarum Grata Voluptas*: Pleasures and Dangers of the Baths', *Proceedings of the British School at Rome*, n.s. 44 (1989), 35–7.

> The tide of ordure that laps at the feet of Roman civilization is simultaneously physical ... and moral. The aediles maintained symbolic as well as literal purity.[78]

The haunts of pleasure – places for drinking, eating, and commercial sex – not blocked sewers or leaking aqueducts, are the places that, as Seneca has it, 'fear the aedile'.[79] And, on Andrew Wallace-Hadrill's seductive reconstruction, the power of élite ideology could translate into a progressive zoning of a city such as Pompeii (and by implication others less well known) so that immoral and thus polluting occupations were excluded from the city's dignified public spaces. In such a moral topography the bath – abode of Venus as well as Hygieia – held a suitably ambiguous position. In Pompeii,

> the façade of the Stabian baths looks nobly onto that part of the Via dell'Abbondanza which seems to have a special status; the back entrance leads within a few yards to the biggest brothel in town.[80]

Such means of purifying urban space were not the preserve of antiquity and the Middle Ages. 'With the onset of a terrible epidemic ... the ... senate passed two decrees intended to clear particular quarters of the city of the beggars infesting them.' The first decree seemed wholly dedicated to placating the deity's wrath, of which the epidemic was an unmistakable sign. 'It strove to create three regions of special holiness, like powerhouses of piety spaced at intervals across the city.' The senate was Venetian, not Roman; the year, 1630.[81] The three regions lay respectively around the doge's chapel – St Mark's – the symbolic centre of the city; around the church of San Rocco, the relevant patron saint; and around the cathedral of San Pietro di Castello.

> In all three holy places the sacrament was to be exposed for adoration and to be accompanied at intervals around the immediate neighbourhood, as though its effluvia were being sent forth to combat the insidious force of the plague.[82]

---

[78]   A. Wallace-Hadrill, 'Public Honour and Private Shame: The Urban Texture of Pompeii', in T.J. Cornell and K. Lomas (eds), *Urban Society in Roman Italy* (London, 1995), p. 51. See also R. Laurence, *Roman Pompeii: Space and Society* (London and New York, 1994), ch. 5. On aediles and public health, O.F. Robinson, *Ancient Rome: City Planning and Administration* (London, 1992), pp. 118–26.

[79]   *On the Truly Happy Life*, 7.3.

[80]   Wallace-Hadrill, 'Public Honour', p. 55.

[81]   B. Pullan, 'Plague and Perceptions of the Poor in Early Modern Italy', in Slack and Ranger, *Epidemics and Ideas*, pp. 101–2. For 'moral sanitation' as a medieval response to plague, in Venice and Florence, see A.G. Carmichael, *Plague and the Poor in Renaissance Florence* (Cambridge, 1986), pp. 98–9, 125.

[82]   Pullan, 'Plague', p. 102.

The boards of magistrates charged with suppressing blasphemy, gambling and other forms of loose living were reminded to do their duty. And, as decreed, the polluting poor were moved on.

Conclusion: secularisation?

All this happened at a time when public health officials and priests had already often come into conflict in Renaissance Italian cities, chiefly on the question of whether the spiritual benefits of processions outweighed the enhanced risk of contagion.[83] So it might seem that, although ritual remained integral to public health in early modern Venice, there had been a good deal of secularisation in perceptions of the subject since classical times. Snapshots of the history of processions across a millennium could be offered as supporting evidence. First exposure: when Pope Gregory the Great ordained a procession in sixth-century Rome, the fact that eighty participants dropped dead was apparently in no way to his discredit. Rather than suggesting that processions enhanced contagion, it proved the urgent necessity for them. Second exposure: when the Black Death reached Avignon, some 750 years later, Pope Clement VI showed himself a true medical pluralist. He banned processions of flagellants, but not on medical grounds; rather, because of their revolutionary zeal. The pope granted indulgences to clergy ministering to the dying, and he instituted a special mass to implore an end to the epidemic. Severe measures were, however, also taken to limit contagion, and physicians were hired to care for the sick.[84] In 1630, by contrast, the year of those Venetian purifications – third exposure – Pope Urban VIII (the one who set the Inquisition on Galileo) responded to a torrent of clerical complaints about secular interference in processions and liturgies by excommunicating the entire Florentine health office.[85] The medical and the religious conceptions of public health were by then distinguishable, as they do not seem to have been in antiquity or for much of the Middle Ages.

Even without the benefit of such snapshots, the history of public health in the West has conventionally been conceived in terms of a sequence of more or less progressive stages. Stage one: Rome, setting the standard. Stage two: the environmental regulations of European cities from 1250 or even earlier (sometimes prompting the suggestion that health as a public good was a

[83]   Palmer, 'The Church, Leprosy and Plague', pp. 95–9; J. Henderson, 'The Black Death in Florence: Medical and Communal Responses', in Bassett, *Death in Towns*, p. 144.
[84]   G. Mollat, *The Popes at Avignon 1305–1378* (London, 1963), pp. 40–41.
[85]   C.M. Cipolla, *Faith, Reason and the Plague* (Sussex, 1979), p. 6.

novelty at the time).[86] Stage three: the segregation of lepers. Stage four: the secularist plague measures of the Italian city-states. Stage five: Enlightened medical 'police'. Then, stimulated by industrialisation, stage six: modern public health, the concept and the administrative category with which we are still familiar.

It could appear that adding the religious dimension to this account of the origins of modern social hygiene would leave the overall evolution intact. The gap in the narrative between the Roman empire and the Italian city-states would be reassuringly filled. And the medieval to early modern phase of the story would then be one not so much of development *ex nihilo* but instead, perhaps, of a slow 'separation of powers', a process which the history of plague measures has been taken to illustrate vividly.[87] Sophisticating the narrative in this way obviously has much to be said in its favour. Yet is doing so quite enough? According to legend, the ancient philosopher Empedocles had the course of two rivers altered to purify a third one, the emanations from which were poisoning the citizens of Selinus. His success was so complete that the citizens acclaimed him as a god – to confirm them in which he leapt, alas fatally, into the flames of Mount Etna.[88] The legend anticipates Hocart. In the beginning, it seems to say, public health is very much to do with the sacred; its officials seem god-like. Yet public health is also depicted in the very practical terms of civil engineering, pretensions to real divinity being dramatically punctured. The religious and the material are already intertwined.

Ancient anecdotes such as that one, no less than the other sources that I have been looking at – Jewish, Roman, Frankish and Venetian – imply that the story of public health cannot altogether be told in simple linear terms. Its religious and ritual aspects resist being confined to the earlier Middle Ages. They do not belong exclusively to a gloomy interlude in a chronicle of otherwise growing enlightenment. They are evident at the story's very beginning. And recent clinical studies suggest that secularism has not yet quite triumphed. Apparently 'religion is good for you', both mentally and physically; one controlled experiment even found that the prayer of others may benefit hospitalised heart patients unaware of the intercession. Like historians, perhaps, 'public health

---

[86]   L. García-Ballester, 'Changes in the *Regimina Sanitatis*: the Role of the Jewish Physicians', in S. Campbell et al. (eds), *Health, Disease and Healing in Medieval Culture* (Basingstoke and London, 1992), p. 120; R.E. Zupko and R.A. Laures, *Straws in the Wind: Medieval Urban Environmental Law – The Case of Northern Italy* (Boulder, CO, and Oxford, 1996).
[87]   Arrizabalaga, 'Facing the Black Death', pp. 250–51.
[88]   Diogenes Laertius, *Lives of the Eminent Philosophers*, 8.70. For context, J. Bidez, *La Biographie d'Empédocle* (Ghent, 1894, repr. 1973).

professionals will have to re-examine long-held assumptions regarding the appropriate roles of science and faith in matters of health'.[89]

---

[89]   For an introduction to the now substantial literature on the 'epidemiology of religion' see J.S. Levin et al., 'Religious Involvement, Health Outcomes, and Public Health Practice', *Current Issues in Public Health*, 2 (1996), 220–25; my final quotation is from p. 223. Also valuable is J. Gartner, 'Religious Commitment, Mental Health, and Prosocial Behavior: a Review of the Empirical Literature', in E.P. Shafranske (ed.), *Religion and the Clinical Practice of Psychology* (Washington, DC, 1996), pp. 187–214.

3

Languages of plague in early modern France

Colin Jones

Historians in general – and medical historians in particular – have tended to be unabashed realists when it comes to bubonic plague.[1] They want to get quickly behind the scanty, skimpy and sometimes misleading texts which deal with the disease in early modern Europe, and get to grips with the big social and epidemiological questions: how was the disease transmitted? How many victims did it carry off? How was it dealt with? How did it end? These are important issues, which require serious attention – and serious answers. In this chapter, however, I wish to essay a different approach, which runs largely counter to current historical practice in plague studies. I have two main aims, both of them very straightforward and simple. First, I wish to suggest that writings on plague in the early modern period, which historians are generally prone to plunder indiscriminately in their quest to determine what actually happened in plague epidemics, often had an internal consistency and a rhetorical structure which make them a significantly flawed source for the social and epidemiological history of the disease. Second, I will argue that historians of plague have tended to underestimate the importance of the languages used about plague in shaping reactions not only to the disease but also to a whole array of problems perceived to be linked to or analogous to it. I suggest, in other words, that we should, on the one hand, be far more cautious

---

[1]   The historiography is simply too vast to be more than evoked. Currently, the finest works of synthesis do not cover France: see P. Slack's classic *The Impact of Plague in Tudor and Stuart England* (London, 1985) and A. Carmichael, *Plague and the Poor in Renaissance Florence* (Cambridge, 1986). For France, see the demographic analyses of J.N. Biraben, *Les Hommes et la peste en France et dans les pays européens et méditerranéens* (2 vols.; Paris, 1975-6), and the social-historical approaches of F. Hildesheimer, *La Terreur et la pitié: L'Ancien Régime à l'épreuve de la peste* (Paris, 1990) and M. Lucenet, *Les Grandes Pestes en France* (Paris, 1985). For an account which tries to mix social with cultural history, see L. Brockliss and C. Jones, *The Medical World of Early Modern France* (Oxford, 1997), esp. chs. 1, 6. I have ventured further down the cultural-historical path in my 'Plague and its metaphors in early modern France', *Representations*, 53 (1996), 97–127, on which the current chapter draws.

about accepting at face value the languages of plague; but that on the other we should be more open to the permeation of those languages in the wider society. This will involve us believing what contemporary texts have to say about plague *less*, but looking to accept, and investigating their influence in society *more*. The focus of the chapter will be on early modern France, but there is every reason for thinking that the approach may be replicated for other societies.

There is no way around plague for the historians of health and medicine, morbidity and mortality, in early modern France. Jean-Noel Biraben has calculated, for example, that between two and two and a half million people died from the disease between 1600 and 1670 alone, making it the largest single cause of adult mortality.[2] No one lived in early modern France, we can wager, without having a friend, neighbour or relative die of the disease. And die horribly, in a polychromatic and explosive cascade of vivid bodily fluids. And die swiftly too: maybe 80 per cent died within a few days of presenting symptoms. Plague, recorded one chronicler, 'has no tomorrows'.[3] In a twinkling of an eye, plague turned the quick into the dead. Throughout the sixteenth century and down to the last third of the seventeenth century, the disease had a massive demographic profile. It went into remission in France in the 1670s, only to reappear in 1720 in the explosion of the disease in Marseilles, half of whose 90,000 population it killed. Massively mortiferous to the end, then, the disease lived on if not in the bodies, at least in the minds and imaginations, the fears and anxieties of French men and women well into the eighteenth century.[4]

An entrée into understanding the cultural resonance of bubonic plague can be made through analysis of the copious literature on plague – printed treatises on the plague, but also other related forms of printed materials ranging from advertisements for quack cures to secret remedies, lists of plague prayers, disputations on knotty academic points, municipal decrees, through to personal memoirs of particular plague attacks.[5] The most extensive and formal of these documents are the treatises on the plague – they are often called something like

---

[2]   Biraben, *Les Hommes et la peste*, 1, pp. 306–10.

[3]   G. Potel, *Traité de la peste advenue en cette ville de Paris, les années 1596 et 1597 et année 1606–1607, comme aussi en l'année 1619* (Paris, 1623), p. 123.

[4]   C. Carrière, M. Coudurié and F. Rebuffat, *Marseille, ville morte* (Marseille, 1968) remains the best account of the last great plague of Western European history. Plague was confined to the Marseilles lazaretto, and prevented from entering the city, on more than a dozen occasions all through the eighteenth century, maintaining the disease at the forefront of contemporaries' minds: D. Panzac, *Quarantaines et lazarets: L'Europe de la peste d'Orient (XVIIe–XXe siècles)* (Aix-en-Provence, 1986), pp. 34ff, 53, 85.

[5]   This is a source on which I have drawn in Jones, 'Plague and its metaphors': p. 103 for a graph showing the chronology of plague literature production between the sixteenth and late eighteenth centuries.

Tractatus Pestis or *traité de la peste*. They offer compendious treatment of the natural history and cultural parameters of the disease: causes of plague; signs and symptoms; the course of the disease; its treatment; how to clean up afterwards.

Although historians have drawn on these documents, they have done so spasmodically and in an unsystematic way, very often aiming to effect a calculus of victims or to ferret out of them examples of 'effective' treatment (usually taken to be quarantines or cordons sanitaires). To my knowledge, there is no comprehensive, nor even semi-comprehensive, listing of these texts for a European country in the early modern period, yet they were extremely numerous and widespread. Drawing on a number of sources, I have been able to list over 250 of them published in France between 1500 and 1770. A good proportion of these were written by ecclesiastics; a similar amount by medical men of varying ilk; the others were largely penned by administrators of various descriptions. These texts are – it must be said, if only to forewarn potential researchers – extremely boring, indeed quite stupendously tedious, and almost wholly bereft of literary merit: 'conventional and derivative' is Paul Slack's description of their English analogues.[6] Daniel Defoe was the shining exception, not the rule.[7] Their endless repetitiveness, their apparent formlessness, plus the fact that large sections of them consist of remedies which were almost without exception useless, makes them seem utterly rebarbative.

Treated with patience and perseverance, however, recurrent patterns of meaning – forms of intertextuality, suggesting a complex of meanings and influences – begin to emerge. By interrogating the literary character and the rhetorical purposes of these texts, one begins to get a sense of a range of purposes implicit within them. At first sight, one suspects the existence of some plague Ur-text – maybe Gregory of Tours, maybe Boccaccio – which was being endlessly repeated and endlessly embroidered upon. The material proves simply too complex and too extensive, however, for any one simple line of genealogy to be recognised.

Plague treatises endlessly purport to offer descriptions of plague epidemics and, indeed, that is why and how historians have seen fit to use them. Yet this descriptive element appears in nearly all cases to be subordinate to a more prescriptive logic or rather logics, for there appear to be at work within the plague texts not one but three scripts for plague, if I can call them that, often overlapping and intercutting amongst themselves. The three scripts for plague correspond in some degree to the trifold characteristics of their authors

---

[6]   Slack, *The Impact of Plague*, p. 24.

[7]   Defoe's powerful *Journal of the Plague Year* told the story of London's last great plague outbreak in 1665 precisely as the last great plague in French history was still in the process of unravelling (1721).

(medics, ecclesiastics and administrators). All, moreover, operate with much the same symbolic system, orientated around the metaphor of the body – a body whose bounds plague has cruelly violated.

	Source	Addressee	Response	Remedy	Objective
Medical	Physician	Patient	Preservation	Regimen	Bodily integrity/ good health
Religious	Ecclesiastic	Christian	Propitiation	Living & dying 'well'	Spiritual integrity/ salvation
Political	Magistrate	Citizen/ subject	Exclusion	Police	Communal integrity/ prosperity

Figure 3.1: Three scripts for plague

Source: C. Jones, 'Plague and its Metaphors in Early Modern France', *Representations*, 53 (1996), 97–127.

In the *medical* script, the argument is addressed to the victim of the disease or would-be patient, and describes the preternatural sensorial assault which plague conducted on the human body, whose integument was visibly almost ripped asunder by exploding buboes, gushing bodily fluids and cadaverous stenches (all described in loving detail). The plague, as the much-republished Guy de Chauliac stated, is 'the prototype of inhumanity', and the human shape and personality become almost unrecognisable under the disease's assault.[8] In the *religious* script, in contrast, arguments are addressed to the body of the faithful. The focus of interest for ecclesiastics in a plague attack was less the atomised biological body ripped asunder, than the collective corpus of believers violated, and losing the spiritual framework within which a Christian life should be lived: as punishment for sin, God sent down a thunderbolt which has penetrated the spiritual carapace of the religious collectivity. Throughout, there is an emphasis on the description of what we could call liturgical violation: church services stop, collective prayers and processions die out; church bells no longer ring out 'the church's time'; the line between the sacred and the profane is blurred; individuals die without receiving last rites and without proper burial

---

[8]   Chauliac is cited in R. Besard, *Discours de la peste* (Dôle, 1630), p. 13.

services.[9] Finally, the *administrative* or *political* script is addressed to the citizen and/or the subject. Authors who are municipal administrators and magistrates are haunted by a different kind of nightmare: less the biological body or the community of saints disrupted than the ruin of the civic life of the collectivity. The bounds of the city are broken as everyone rushes to leave; organised trade stops; shops close; crime and looting abounds; the boundaries of the private and the public break down; hierarchy is no longer respected; even family bonds count for nothing, as mothers abandon their babies, children their parents; everything is out of place.

The three scripts for plague which one can detect pulsating and interweaving through the plague literature offer three nightmares, then, three almost carnivalesquely dystopic visions of what plague can do. Yet one person's dystopia is another's utopia. Besides presenting a vision of the world turned upside down, the plague texts also have a strongly prescriptive dimension. They show the body violated, but also offer a vision of the stricken body being reintegrated and healed, of the boundaries of the violated body being reinstated.

This restorative logic is apparent in each of the three scripts. Purely *medical* texts may include a range of remedies and prescriptions, for example, though the best-founded medical knowledge urges self-preservation rather than cure as a means of restoring and/or maintaining bodily integrity and good health. Medical literature orients the patient around observation of a stout regimen: to prevent the bodies bursting their bounds, one should live moderately well – no boozing, no gluttony, moderate physical exercise, not too much (maybe no) sexual intercourse, and so on – according to the time-honoured respect for the non-naturals. In the *religious* script, the way to achieve spiritual integrity for the communion of saints, and salvation for the individual believer, in contrast, is seen as coming through spiritual propitiation. God must be appeased for mankind's sin: in prayer and penance lies the way towards spiritual wholeness. The continuity of liturgy should be ensured through the continued presence of the clergy in the plague-stricken locality. When in 1576 Saint Charles Borromeo, Archbishop of Milan, had stayed among his flock in the middle of a plague epidemic, he set an exemplar for clerical conduct which transcended the much-followed advice available to the social and religious élite: *cito, longe, tarde* ('leave early, go far, come back late'). The horrid death in a plague epidemic – unshriven, sudden, anonymous; victims dying in the gutter, dumped unceremoniously into mass graves – was the antithesis of the 'good death' diffused by Counter-Reformation piety.[10] The ecclesiastic plague text was thus

---

[9]   J. Le Goff, 'Merchant's time and church's time in the Middle Ages' in *idem*, *Time, War and Culture in the Middle Ages* (Chicago, 1980), pp. 29–42.

[10]   For the literature of the 'good death', see R. Chartier, 'Les Arts de mourir, 1450–1600' and D. Roche, 'La Mémoire de la mort: recherche sur la place des arts de mourir dans la

a pedagogic, pastoral, maybe even propagandising document, a religious tool within an overarching strategy of Christianisation. The dystopic vision of the plague served only to enhance the picture of a putative piety for the true believer.

If the utopian vision of the religious plague text was a community of saints ensuring spiritual rectitude and liturgical continuity, the *administrative* text for plague had similarly prescriptive intent. The image of the community breaking down under the presence of disease is countered by an increasingly elaborate set of administrative procedures: ones, moreover, pretty familiar to historians. The litany is gradually established: clear the streets, clean the drains, remove rubbish, police the markets, kill cats and dogs, expel beggars, close brothels, organise food supply, man the city gates, supervise trade and circulation, employ medical staff and orderlies, open the infirmaries for the sick, light bonfires, shoot off cannons, introduce quarantines, and think about a cordon sanitaire. The model for this new version of civic virtue is that of the well-administered, well-run polity, its magistrates faithfully at their posts. Most often, this is seen in terms of city government. As the seventeenth century wears on, however, it is also seen in terms of the central government. Just as, we may surmise, the religious plague text exemplifies the Christianising strategies of the post-Tridentine Catholic church, so the administrative plague text serves the interests and furbishes the image of Bourbon absolutism.[11]

It would seem, therefore, that the plague text was emphatically more interesting and revealing that its innocent, arid, infra-literary text character appears to suggest. Pulsating within it were a set of sometimes complementary, sometimes competing programmes for action. This should make historians far more wary of reading them as unproblematic reflections of, or comments on, an anterior and pre-existent reality. Maybe plague texts can give us a sense of what 'actually happened' in plague outbreaks, 'how it really was' to adopt a Rankean terminology. More important, I would argue, is to understand what was going on in these texts. Descriptive passages are always under the severe cautions of a set of latent rhetorical purposes. Indeed, if we accept the argument that the plague texts often utilise the image of the plague with other ends in mind, then we can accept the possibility that they might exaggerate the impact of the disease. This, indeed, seems very likely: in plague epidemics, deaths routinely ascribed to plague were often due to other causes; medically qualified searchers and gravediggers were hardly trustworthy diagnosticians; deaths from

---

librairie et la lecture en France aux XVIIe et XVIIIe siècles', *Annales. Économies. Sociétés. Civilisations*, 31 (1976), 76–119.

[11]   This, of course, is Michel Foucault's plague text: see his *Discipline and Punish: The Birth of the Prison* (London, 1979), pp. 195–8. Though brilliantly highlighting what I have called the administrative script for plague, Foucault underestimates, I would contend, the internal complexity and the plurality of plague scenarios.

fevers and other illnesses could be put at plague's door; all deaths in hospitals, lazarettos, plague-infected households were similarly ascribed; and there were cases, too, of sick individuals being sewn screaming into shrouds before being carted off to plague pits. So, too, we can be demographically fairly certain that even if we took all deaths in time of plague as plague deaths, the latter would still pale in comparison with childhood deaths, about which physicians, churchmen and administrators are relatively silent. Probably more than five times as many children died before their first birthday in early modern France, than died of bubonic plague. Infant mortality might have won any retrospective body-count race; but it lacked plague's cultural resonance, its ability to stand as 'the prototype of inhumanity'.[12]

We might indeed go further than this, and seek to reverse the terms of historians' usual approach to these texts. Rather than the texts providing a transparent window onto a reality 'out there', maybe that reality was, in fact, constructed by the competing cultural logics implicit in such texts. We therefore need to consider the extent to which the script offered in the plague texts was a script that was actually enacted. In order to come to terms with such an approach, we require a print history of these texts which will allow us to gauge their influence. Which were the most important? Which circulated most widely? Which were printed and reprinted – and plagiarised? Who read them? How does what they recommend and prescribe meet up with what was actually done on the ground? What were the social – as opposed to the textual – consequences of the construction of disease in these writings?[13] All these are questions which historians have scarcely thought of asking – let alone answering.

It is bubonic plague's ability to carry hefty symbolic freight which I would like to evoke in conclusion. Plague – *la peste* – came to signify in early modern France almost any kind of pestilence, epidemiological disaster, noxious prodigy or human catastrophe.[14] Indeed, whereas historians have devoted much of their energy to questions considering the contagiousness (or otherwise) of bubonic plague, they have missed the extent to which discourses on plague infected a whole range of other languages: the language of plague was perhaps more contagious than plague itself. We could follow this inference in the medical and the religious worlds, but let us take, by way of example, its dissemination in languages of state. The victory over plague was very largely perceived as a victory for the administrative script for plague which had been sketched out in

---

[12]   Jones, 'Plague and its metaphors', n. 25 for the statistics.

[13]   This would follow in the tracks of the works of H.-J. Martin, R. Chartier, R. Darnton et al. For a primer, see the multi-volumed H.-J. Martin and R. Chartier (eds), *Histoire de l'édition française* (Paris, 1983–86) 4 vols.

[14]   A.M. Brenot, 'La peste soit des Huguenots: étude d'une logique d'exécration au XVIe siècle', *Histoirie, économie, société*, 11 (1992), 553–70.

plague treatises, and it redounded very largely to the credit of the state. Plague was viewed as having been essentially conquered by the cordon sanitaire, the elevation to the national and even international scale, of measures of segregation and distancing which had been utilised empirically by individual localities since the fourteenth century. We see this in the success of the campaign to keep the Normandy plague of 1665–67 out of Paris – a movement which was personally engineered by the king's principal minister, Colbert – and in the similarly effective campaign to contain plague in the environs of Marseilles in 1720.[15]

Yet the victory for the enactment of the prescriptive administrative discourse to be found in plague treatises also influenced the way in which a wide range of social and cultural problems were viewed in late seventeenth- and early eighteenth-century France. The language of the plague containment was also in fact the language of the 'Great Confinement of the Poor', the movement to institutionalise the poor and the deviant in special institutions, or 'general hospitals'. Beggars, vagrants, prostitutes, gypsies, delinquents, recalcitrant Protestants, lunatics, all were regarded as being a kind of contagious yeast which needed to be kept under control – normally this came to mean institutionalisation.[16] The flora and fauna of the worlds of poverty, deviance and vice were construed as being as contagious as a plague victim, his or her bodily boundedness grotesquely burst asunder. Thus, one writer in 1607 equated a pauper with a plague victim,

> noteworthy by a conspicuous rash, mange, itch, canker; bleeding with ulcers and scrofulas; hobbled, covered with boils and pus, epileptic, leprous, all wounded, deformed and horrible in their visages; all but skin and bone, like flayed corpses, in whom we see the veins and the nerves all uncovered; and so stunted and puny that one can remark their entrails moving within their breasts.[17]

Today, historians of medicine might well regard questions relating to poverty and the Great Confinement as beyond their remit. Certainly, the latter had none of the retrospective lustre of the campaigns to eradicate plague. Yet, if we wish to understand the meaning of plague in early modern society, we will need to understand some of these linkages. And in so doing, we should

---

[15] Brockliss and Jones, *The Medical World*, esp. pp. 350–56. For a triumphalist eighteenth-century account, see J. Sénac and M. Chicoyneau, *Traité des causes, des accidents et de la cure de la peste, avec un recueil d'observations* (Paris, 1744).

[16] The classic account is M. Foucault, *Folie et déraison, Histoire de la folie à l'âge classique* (Paris, 1961). Cf. Brockliss and Jones, *The Medical World*, esp. ch. 11.

[17] *La Chimère ou Phantosme de la mendicité* (n.p., 1607), 2.

stray beyond plague texts simply to estimate a calculus of suffering; we will also need to understand the cultural logics implicit within them and the way they resonated more broadly within the wider society.

4

Copenhagen 1711: Danish authorities facing the plague

Peter Christensen

The problem

In late 1708, the Danish government received warning of a major outbreak of plague approaching from the south. Originating, apparently, in the Ottoman empire, the plague had crossed the Balkans and then spread into Central and Eastern Europe. By autumn 1708 it had reached Poland. The following year it spread to Pomerania, east Prussia and Lithuania and then proceeded to engulf the entire Baltic region. By late November 1710 Lübeck, just across the Holstein border, had been infected and a few weeks later the plague was reported to be ravaging Sweden. At that time, Denmark, arrayed with Russia, Poland and Saxony, was waging the Great Northern War to break Sweden's domination of the Baltic and to recover the lost land of Scania. Fighting ranged from Bremen eastwards far into the Ukraine. Military movements and the resulting disorder facilitated the progress of the plague. The mortality of the outbreak was severe. Between 1709 and 1711 the plague killed a third of the population of East Prussia and Brandenburg. Lithuania is said to have suffered even greater mortality, losing 40 per cent of the population to the disease. Sweden was badly hit as well: in Stockholm 30 per cent of the inhabitants died.[1]

Evolution of a solution

It is commonly assumed that plague, after its initial appearance in the fourteenth century, gradually reduced in ferocity and eventually became a predominantly urban phenomenon.[2] This may be true of England, but the

---

[1]   M. Vasold, *Pest, Not und schwere Plagen. Seuchen und Epidemien vom Mittelalter bis heute* (München, 1991), pp. 168–69; G. Sticker, *Abhandlungen aus der Seuchengeschichte und Seuchenlehre* (Giessen, 1908–1912), 1 (1908), p. 216.
[2]   See, for example, R. Gottfried, *The Black Death: Natural and Human Disaster in*

general validity of these views is not confirmed by the 1708–13 outbreak which ravaged both the towns and the countryside of Eastern and Central Europe with unabated virulence. With few exceptions, Danish historians working on medieval and early modern periods have been Malthusians. An overview of the literature published in recent decades shows implicitly that plague and other epidemic diseases are consistently seen as by-products of subsistence crises and therefore of little intrinsic interest. Thus, the history of plague in Denmark remains somewhat obscure. It seems, however, that morbidity conformed to the general European pattern and after the initial outbreak in 1348–51, at least twenty major outbreaks are recorded. Though the fourteenth and fifteenth centuries in particular are poorly documented, all Danish plagues seem to have been parts of larger, transregional epidemics, chiefly originating in the Baltic.[3] Severe outbreaks originating there spread to Denmark in 1604–5, in the early 1620s, in 1629 and again in 1636–37.

Denmark, like most other European countries, had become accustomed to the plague and had developed a number of routine precautionary measures against the disease. The first line of defence included efforts to prevent contact with infected areas outside the country and that primarily meant the Baltic. Thus in 1653, when plague was once more spreading round the Baltic, the Danish authorities put heavy restrictions on trade and travel to the infected ports. These restrictions were not lifted until the following spring but this turned out to be premature. A Dutch grain ship from Danzig brought the plague to Copenhagen, where 30 per cent of the population died during the summer. Efforts to contain the disease failed and it spread to most parts of Denmark, eventually reaching Norway. Again, in the late 1650s when Denmark was desperately fighting for its survival as an independent state, plague was spread in Jutland, this time apparently by Polish troops.

Once peace was restored, and Denmark had become an absolutist state, the authorities made measures stricter and more detailed. When plague was reported in the Low Countries in 1663 all imports from there and from Hamburg were banned. Nobody was permitted to go ashore from the ships arriving from these places and soldiers were stationed in the ports to ensure compliance. Again, in August 1665 when plague was reported in London, orders were issued that all goods and passengers from England were to be quarantined, even if they were carrying health certificates. Similar measures were adopted in the autumn of 1680 when plague was ravaging Germany, though this time travellers with valid health certificates were allowed to enter Denmark.[4] Neither

Medieval Europe (London, 1983); M.W. Flinn, *The European Demographic System, 1500–1820* (Brighton, 1981), pp. 51–2.

[3]   J.H. Ibs, 'Die Pest in Schleswig-Holstein von 1350 bis 1547/48', *Kieler Werkstücke, Reihe A: Beiträge zur schleswig-holsteinischen und skandinavischen Geschichte* (1994).

[4]   O. Nielsen (ed.), *Kjøbenhavns Diplomatarium*, vols 1–8 (København, 1872–1887), 6,

of these two major European outbreaks reached Denmark. Thus, by the late seventeenth century Denmark was apparently able to prevent infection.

The 1711 outbreak

When plague was reported in Poland in 1708, the Danish government began applying the customary precautionary measures: health certificates were demanded of all ships returning from the Baltic, suspicious ships were to be quarantined for forty days and all letters from the area were to be thoroughly fumigated.[5] In November 1710, when the plague had moved closer, reaching Lübeck, the chief of the Copenhagen police was instructed to register all travellers and inquire into their origin, their business, and how long they intended to stay. All of which was to be done on specially printed forms, distributed by the police.[6] Soon after, when plague was reported in Sweden, health certificates were made mandatory for everybody travelling within the kingdom and these certificates were to be issued free of any charge. In particular, the inhabitants of Saltholmen (a small island outside Copenhagen) were forbidden on pain of death to enter Copenhagen without certificates and under no circumstances were they to have any contact with Scania just across the Sound.[7] The authorities also stepped up their usual efforts to make the city cleaner. Citizens were forbidden to dump refuse and rubbish in the streets or to raise animals inside the city, in particular unclean pigs, which might cause disease-producing miasmas. Considering how often these orders were repeated, it would seem that no progress was made.[8]

This time the precautionary measures proved insufficient. In March 1711 plague had definitely appeared in the small, busy sea port of Helsingør (Elsinore), 20 miles north of Copenhagen. It was most likely brought by soldiers from the army fighting in Sweden or by sailors from the navy operating in the Baltic. The local community attempted to conceal plague deaths and as a result, soldiers were sent to seal off the town, rather belatedly to be effective. They were ordered to shoot to kill anyone trying to leave and were backed up by warships stationed offshore to control the approach by sea. When the

---

pp. 391, 403, 409, 744.
[5]   Nielsen, *Kjøbenhavns Diplomatarium*, 8, p. 48.
[6]   Nielsen, *Kjøbenhavns Diplomatarium*, 8, pp. 133–4.
[7]   Nielsen, *Kjøbenhavns Diplomatarium*, 8, pp. 138–9, 135.
[8]   Sv. Cedergreen Bech, *Københavns Historie* (Copenhagen, 1967), pp. 250–51; see also *Kancelliets Brevbøger* (1584–88), p. 760, for earlier, unsuccessful efforts in this direction. Copenhagen did in fact have a sort of organised refuse (and night soil) removal, but the private entrepreneurs who ran this were not known for efficiency. On the other hand, the entrepreneurs constantly complained that the citizens, 'even those of noble extraction' were not really being co-operative.

outbreak had run its course the small town had lost 40 per cent of its inhabitants.[9] In Copenhagen, the police received strict orders to inquire if anybody had arrived from Helsingør and to inspect all corpses before burial.[10] Yet the plague evaded the delayed isolation efforts, probably thanks to military movements, and appeared in the capital in June. It seems initially that the medical authorities were somewhat reluctant to recognise the first suspicious cases, perhaps because they knew how the plague regulations would disrupt life in the city. By July, however, there was no doubt.[11] Wealthy citizens began to flee the city and the authorities put into force an additional number of well-tried measures to prevent further spread of the disease.

First, a day of nationwide prayer was ordered.[12] Second, the university was instructed to produce cheap books on how to prevent and cure plague. This was standard procedure in times of plague and the effort usually consisted of the reprinting of older tracts.[13] The advice and cures offered were, of course, quite useless, but the order may serve as an indication of how the authorities sought to use the fairly high literacy level of Denmark to promote public health. Third, and most importantly, attempts were made at quickly isolating sources of infection inside Copenhagen. In the final analysis, no doubt, the appearance of plague was to be considered a punishment from God, but the authorities had long ago drawn the conclusion that transmission of the disease occurred through contagion. Isolation of diseased individuals and infected objects, particularly clothing and linen, were essential procedures. A special Health Commission, consisting of civil servants such as the chief of police and the Medical Officer of Health, and a number of prominent citizens, was set up to assist the authorities in containing the disease.[14] Wodroffsgård, a large estate outside Copenhagen, was rented to serve as a plague isolation hospital. Later, the military hospital (in spite of the protests of the army) and a royal estate were also commandeered.[15] It quickly became clear that the old cemeteries of Copenhagen, including the cemetery attached to the original plague hospital, were insufficient. In July, the Commission therefore established a large new cemetery outside Østerport (the eastern gate) where, it seems, the majority of

---

[9]   F.V. Mansa, 'Pesten i Kjøbenhavn', *Historisk Tidsskrift*, 1 (1840), 414.

[10]   Nielsen, *Kjøbenhavns Diplomatarium*, 8, p. 157.

[11]   The symptoms were described by Dr Mule: see C. Mule (ed.), *Kjøbenhavn under Pesten 1711. Samtidige Breve* (Copenhagen, 1843), pp. 306, 317.

[12]   Nielsen, *Kjøbenhavns Diplomatarium*, 8, p. 194.

[13]   Nielsen, *Kjøbenhavns Diplomatarium*, VI, pp. 744–5.

[14]   The authorities in Copenhagen appointed a Medical Officer of Health (Stadsphysicus) around 1625, though he was paid only in times of plague. Not until 1699 was the post turned into a regular, salaried office.

[15]   Nielsen, *Kjøbenhavns Diplomatarium*, 8, pp. 158, 181, 183–4. Like other European cities, Copenhagen used to have a special plague hospital, but it had been destroyed in the siege of 1659. As there had not been any plague after that, the hospital was never rebuilt.

poor plague victims were buried. The Commission also had the foresight to establish a temporary orphanage. The police force was increased to enforce the plague regulations.[16] Nobody could enter or leave the city without a health certificate, and only Nørreport (the north gate) would remain open for traffic; vagrants and beggars were to be forcibly rounded up and put in quarantine; all letters sent from Copenhagen were to be fumigated; schools were closed; large congregations were to be avoided and priests were instructed to shorten services.

In addition to these general measures practised in the urban environment, which aimed to prevent plague by policing society, the bodies of plague victims, their immediate effects and personal environment were also subject to additional emergency controls. All suspicious deaths were to be reported immediately. All infected houses were to be sealed off, diseased inhabitants being transferred to the plague hospital, while the healthy went to either a quarantine station for two weeks or remained confined to their house (where they would receive provisions from the Health Commission). Clothes belonging to the deceased persons were to be burned and all trade in used clothes, woollens, bedding and so on was strictly forbidden. Interference with the work of the police was forbidden and contravention of this order was punishable by the death penalty. Plague victims were to be buried within 24 hours. Only specially appointed bearers could handle corpses. Special hearses and biers were used and funeral processions were forbidden. Free coffins were provided for the poor.

The Health Commission was instructed to ensure equitable distribution of provisions inside the city. Food riots were not to obstruct the isolation efforts.[17] In this, the Commission was successful. However, it was less successful in checking the progress of the plague. It spread inside the city, peaking in August 1711, when 2,400 people died in a single week.[18] Together with convicts from the Bremerholm shipyard, 200 soldiers from the garrison were detailed to dig mass graves for the poor (though actual burial did not take place until the valuable soldiers had done their job and been moved away). But the production of coffins could not keep up with the mortality. The shallow graves in the crowded cemeteries emitted a terrible stench that hung over the city, and the firing of cannons in the cemeteries did little to dispel the tainted air. Not until October, and the beginning of cold weather, did the the plague finally release

---

[16]   H. Matthiessen, 'Fra den Store Pest 1711: Pestkirkegaarden paa Østerbro', *Historiske Meddelelser om København*, 2 rk, 1 (1924), 386–396; Mule, *Kjøbenhavn under Pesten 1711*, p. 306.

[17]   Nielsen, *Kjøbenhavns Diplomatarium*, 8, pp. 163–79, 185–91, 198–201.

[18]   Mansa, 'Pesten i Kjøbenhavn' 4 (1843); E. Marquard, 'En Statistik fra Pestens Aar 1711', *Historiske Meddelelser om København*, 2 rk, 1 (1924), 397–402.

its grip on Copenhagen.[19] By then, plague had been responsible for between 22,000–23,000 deaths among a population of 60,000, most of them poor people. The wealthy, about 5,000 people, had fled the city at the beginning of the epidemic.[20] Restrictions on travel and other activities, however, were not lifted until 22 June 1712, the same day the Commission finally resigned.

Considering the severe mortality it would seem that the efforts of the authorities and of the Health Commission in particular had not been effective. A number of accusations were brought (mostly anonymously) against the Commission for being on the one hand inefficient, and on the other highhanded in dealing with the public. This was largely unjustified. The Commission seems to have worked hard and courageously and did as well as could be expected under the circumstances. Quite apart from the fact that there was no clear consensus concerning the nature of the disease and how it was transmitted, any assessment must take account of the obstacles facing the Commission.[21]

First, the Commission did not have any executive powers. All measures and regulations had to be approved by the king's representatives *outside* Copenhagen and this hindered the already cumbersome bureaucratic procedures. Second, the Commission met with opposition from the guilds and other institutions who resented interference in their work and priorities. The military, in particular – for fear that valuable soldiers might be lost – constantly refused requests and ignored quarantine measures. Third, a complete quarantine could not be enforced as the city had to be provisioned from the outside. And fourthly, there were economic considerations. The Commission had some funding for its work, but valuable resources might be lost by being too zealous. Twice the king insisted that all clothing and linen belonging to deceased persons should be burned, and each time the Commission delayed and protested. Not only did the items represent considerable value by pre-industrial standards, they would also be indispensable to the poor in the approaching winter (after being properly washed and fumigated, of course).[22] Finally, the inhabitants of the plague-stricken city in a number of cases ignored all precautionary measures. Hans Mule, Professor of medicine and a member of the Commission, complained that the populace was an unruly and intractable lot that paid heed neither to laws nor to regulations and did not hesitate to move goods from sealed houses.[23]

---

[19]   Nielsen, *Kjøbenhavns Diplomatarium*, 8, pp. 182, 192. The attempts to safeguard the military were unsuccessful, the garrison of Copenhagen and the navy suffered many plague deaths.

[20]   Mansa, 'Pesten i Kjøbenhavn' 1 (1840); Marquard, 'En Statistik fra Pestens Aar 1711'.

[21]   See Mansa 'Pesten i Kjøbenhavn' (1840–43) for detailed information on the work of the Commission.

[22]   Mule, *Kjøbenhavn under Pesten 1711*, pp. 322, 327.

[23]   Ibid., pp. 303, 318, 320.

Perhaps it was not surprising that the Commission failed to stop the infection from spreading inside Copenhagen. This failure, however, should not overshadow the real successes of the Danish authorities in 1711. For the first time, a major outbreak was contained. Unlike the great epidemics of the 1600s, the 1711 plague did not spread across the entire country: it had become an urban problem. It seems that the government, after the infection of Copenhagen, more or less wrote off the rest of Zealand. Very strict quarantine measures were imposed to save Funen and Jutland, but in fact Zealand did not fare too badly. Besides Copenhagen (and Elsinore) three more towns, all in close contact with the capital, were infected: Hillerød, Køge, and Roskilde. In the first two, infection was said to have been brought by linen and clothing illegally removed from infected and sealed houses in Copenhagen. In Roskilde the mortality was severe (close to 50 per cent), but although some cases were reported from the countryside, Zealand as a whole was spared a major mortality crisis, which was one of the reasons for the rapid recovery of Copenhagen's population.[24] The duchies (that is, Schleswig-Holstein) were also infected, probably by the military, but this outbreak was also checked.[25]

The great enigma

In 1720, when the Great Northern War was over, plague again appeared in the ports of the Baltic. Once more the Danish authorities started all the routine measures and, as in the 1660s and 1680s, they were successful in preventing the infection from reaching Denmark.[26] Seen in this perspective, the outbreak of plague in 1711 had been an unfortunate accident caused by wartime conditions. Even so, the Danish authorities, in the end, managed to contain it. This links the Copenhagen outbreak to the wider issue of what part human action played in the disappearance of the plague. The epidemic of 1708–13 turned out to be the last in Western and Central Europe, but what actually made the plague disappear is often referred to as one of the great enigmas in history.[27] A number of different and sometimes ingenious explanations have been suggested, ranging from rat immunity to improved housing. None of them are really satisfactory.[28] The issue needs to be seen in a broader, comparative perspective. The plague only disappeared from Western and Central Europe. In Eastern

---

[24]   Ibid., pp. 309, 319; Mansa 'Pesten i Kjøbenhavn' (1843), pp. 118–19; Nielsen, *Kjøbenhavns Diplomatarium*, 8, p. 226.

[25]   Mansa 'Pesten i Kjøbenhavn' (1843), pp. 126–7.

[26]   Nielsen, *Kjøbenhavns Diplomatarium*, 8, pp. 503–4.

[27]   P. Slack, 'The Disappearance of Plague: an Alternative View', *Economic History Review*, 34 (1981), 469–76.

[28]   A.B. Appleby, 'The Disappearance of the Plague: a Continuing Puzzle', *Economic History Review* (2nd series) 33 (1980), 161–173.

Europe and the Middle East, outbreaks continued for another century.[29] Obviously, what made the plague decline had to be something particular to Western Europe. It may be that Western and Central Europe enjoyed the special advantage of having no inveterate plague focuses and the use of quarantine must have been the crucial factor. The counter-argument is that quarantine had been put into use for centuries without noticeable effect. The measures adopted by the Danish authorities in the eighteenth century did not differ markedly from those adopted by the Italian city-states in the fourteenth century. But by the second half of the seventeenth century the agency enforcing the quarantine measures had changed, in part as society's response to the constant threat of plague. European states became more powerful. Whether European absolutism was the political apparatus of aristocratic rule or not, it did bring about a consolidation of larger territorial units, a centralisation of government, and an increase and professionalisation of the civil service. In Denmark, in theory the most absolutist state of all, the plague regulations reflect the confidence of the authorities in their ability to deal with crises. On the whole, this confidence was justified. Danish absolutism succeeded in containing plague coming across the Baltic, just as Austrian absolutism succeeded in containing infection from the Ottoman lands. The impressive plague cordon along the southern border of Austria-Hungary was established as a direct result of the 1708–13 epidemic and must rank as the greatest achievement of Habsburg rule.[30] In 1770, when plague again was ravaging Russia and Poland, Prussia established a similar cordon sanitaire, completing the insulation of Central Europe from the plague.

Epidemic disease and recurring mortality crises had been part of civilized society for millennia. The containment of the plague was the first major break with this ancient pattern and it was achieved, not by any marked increase in scientific medical knowledge, but through what were essentially police measures. Michael Flinn called this 'a triumph of human organization'. More correctly, perhaps, it should be considered a triumph of regimentation. During the subsistence crises of the 1740s and 1770s the Danish authorities adopted the same precautionary restrictions on travelling and other activities and thus prevented the large-scale spread of typhus.[31] In 1810, the Danish government took another basic step towards improving general health conditions by making the new technology of smallpox vaccination mandatory for everybody, and

---

[29]   M.W. Dols, 'The Second Plague Pandemic and its Recurrences in the Middle East, 1347–1894', *Journal of the Economic and Social History of the Orient*, 22 (1979), 162–89; D. Panzac, *La Peste dans l'Empire Ottoman, 1700–1850* (Leuven, 1985).

[30]   The cordon did not become fully operational until the mid-eighteenth century, but it did indicate the determination and capability of the absolutist state. See E. Lesky, 'Die österreichische Pestfront an der k.k. Militärgrenze', *Saeculum* (1957), 82–106.

[31]   J.D. Post, 'The Mortality Crisis of the Early 1770s and the European Demographic Trends,' *Journal of Interdisciplinary History*, 21 (1990), 29–62.

using its proven administrative capability to enforce the measure.[32] Even centralistic France was not able to promulgate a corresponding law until a century later.

The record of pre-industrial state intervention in Denmark is fairly impressive. The state successfully regulated trade and banking; it began to organise a system of free schooling and, in the 1780s, defused social conflicts through a series of agrarian reforms. Together with the successful disease control, all of this indicates that the Danish authorities, by the standards of the time, performed more effectively than most of their European counterparts. Seen in a broader, global perspective these differences seem less important, however. What mattered was the singular efforts made by most European states to contain common epidemic diseases. Though these efforts were not based on scientific medical knowledge, they were to a large extent successful and remain a key precondition, if not a direct cause, for the European mortality decline.

---

[32] H. Schou (ed.), *Cronologisk Register over kongelige Forordninger og aabne Breve*, vol. 15 (Copenhagen, 1812), pp. 478–86.

5

Fighting for public health: Dr Duncan and his adversaries, 1847–1863

Paul Laxton

The career of William Henry Duncan offers important connections between the history of health and the history of the city. Indeed, his work was more sharply focused on the correlation between the new form of urban environment and public health than that of almost any other Victorian health reformer. His practical view of public health was applied to, and learned from, the neighbourhoods, streets and courts of Liverpool, where his reputation began and ended. 'The men in authority – in London', he once wrote to the medical officer for Barnsley, 'are theorists, and don't look at the practical or practicable side of the question.'[1] However, to describe and assess the issues, ideologies and individuals that shaped Duncan's period of office as Britain's first full-time medical officer of health, we need to discard the pervading heroic mythology of an enlightened man doing battle with stubborn ignorance and self-interest. Such Whiggism does disservice to medical history, urban history and W.H. Duncan.

Duncan as idol

Duncan has been idolised by the public health professionals, his reputation carefully guarded as the founding father of Liverpool's heroic struggle against the agents of ill health. The most eloquent statement of his public virtues came from the pen of the unrivalled leader among Victorian municipal medical officers, Sir John Simon.[2] It would be wrong to say that his reputation was invented, but it has certainly been given a vigorous spin. The recent (1997)

---

[1] Liverpool Record Office (hereafter LivRO) MOH letter books 3, f. 116. Duncan to Thomas Saddler, 3 October 1860.

[2] J. Simon, *English Sanitary Institutions* (London, 1897) 2nd edn, pp. 246–8.

150th anniversary of Duncan's appointment is a perfect embodiment of what Jacyna has described in the case of John Hunter: for public health to gain the public recognition it undoubtedly needs, it must have an appropriate, packageable past.[3] It needs a mythology. Demythologising heroes need not necessarily be a negative exercise. The case of Florence Nightingale is well known: a heroine for the greater part of her life, whose status as a national icon was largely of her own devising. Yet if she emerges from F.B. Smith's literary autopsy as far from the virtuous illuminator, she now seems a great deal more interesting and no longer beyond the historians' sights.[4] More recently, and with closer relevance to Duncan, Christopher Hamlin's masterly assessment of Edwin Chadwick's role in the creation of the concept of public health challenges the largely unexamined picture of the great architect of sanitary progress. The simple picture of a man beleaguered by vested interests in his fight against obvious problems with clear technical and environmental solutions, misses the political complexity of the issues, but also fails to recognise Chadwick's political cunning based on his own understanding of those complexities.[5] Hamlin draws explicit lessons for modern public health policy: since public health has been a matter of choices, whose past as well as present must be vigorously debated, it will not do for the professionals to draw on an uncontested and tidy past. 'More than in other institutions, driven by the whims of markets or polities, professionals rely for their senses of identity and mission on history. These thorny issues were surely settled definitively at some time in the past, professionals assure themselves; we are thankful we need not undergo the exhausting process of reinventing or rejustifying ourselves'.[6]

It is common enough for reputations to be made only after the death of the subject, but Duncan is interesting partly because he had little public reputation in his lifetime, partly because of the sort of people who *did* regard him highly in his lifetime, and partly for the *reasons* they did. There was no great public funeral (compare James Newlands, the Borough Engineer, who in 1871 received a ceremonious public burial in the Necropolis), death notices in the general and professional press were muted and matter-of-fact, his salary, staff and general status in the corporation were in all respects modest, and his only local memorial is a wall plaque from St Jude's church, Hardwick Street, now displayed in the Liverpool Medical Institution.[7]

---

[3]   L.S. Jacyna 'Images of John Hunter in the nineteenth century', *History of Science*, 21 (1983), 85–108. I am grateful to Dr Helen Power for drawing my attention to this paper.

[4]   F.B. Smith, *Florence Nightingale: Reputation and Power* (London, 1982).

[5]   C. Hamlin, *Public Health and Social Justice in the Age of Chadwick: Britain 1800–1854* (Cambridge, 1998).

[6]   Ibid., p. 340.

[7]   In 1859 when Duncan was paid £750 per annum, the Town Clerk was paid £2,500, Newlands and three other officers £1,000, Thomas Duncan, the Water Engineer, £800, and

It would be interesting to unravel the history of Duncan's reputation, but that is not the main theme of this chapter. It is, however, important to observe that heroes generally need enemies. Routing the opposition is an essential part of being a heroic figure – part of the panegyric; and if the obstacles are human rather than elemental, so much the better. This is the all too familiar 'microbes and men' approach.[8]

Who were the architects of this image, with all its hyperbole? Why has Duncan's name been evoked and used without the slightest inclination on the part of its users to evaluate the man and his work? These questions are beyond the scope of this chapter, but they are an important part of its context. One possible reason why Duncan was far from idolised in his own lifetime was that he found himself (in some cases placed himself) in conflict with too many parties. A public health officer has no obvious body of supporters.

Duncan's career in summary

Born in Liverpool into a well-connected family of merchants in 1805 (nine months before his famous uncle Dr James Currie died), Duncan was educated by another uncle, a Scottish Presbyterian minister in Dumfriesshire, and trained as a physician in Edinburgh, receiving his MD in 1829. After spending some time in France, he set up in practice in Liverpool, served in the hospitals (as physician and lecturer) and voluntary dispensaries, gained something of a reputation in the cholera epidemic of 1832, published his first paper (a statistical study) in 1833, and became secretary to various medical and learned bodies as well as the Liverpool Health of Towns Association. Either on his own volition or by invitation he provided evidence for parliamentary enquiries in 1833, 1836, 1840, 1842 and 1844, in all cases on questions of the relationship between, on the one hand, housing and social conditions and, on the other, the health of the people. Thus, in his thirties he developed a considerable expertise in researching that topic, assembling statistical data, and presenting it in person or in print in trenchant and effective ways. Following his remarkable paper of 1843, *On the physical causes of the high rate of mortality in Liverpool*, which is reproduced with only minor editorial cuts in the first report of the Commission on Large Towns and Populous Districts in 1844, Duncan was the established expert on public health in 'the most unhealthy

---

W.T. McGowen, Chief Assistant to the Town Clerk, £600. *A Return ... of the names, occupations, and salaries of all the officers, clerks, and servants in the employ, or paid by, the Corporation of Liverpool ... on the 31st December, 1859, 1864, and 1869 ...* (Liverpool, 1870).

8   R. Reid, *Microbes and Men* (London, 1974).

town in England' as he called it, and his reputation began to spread abroad.[9] He was a workaholic, an indefatigable assembler of data, obsessive in establishing its correctness, and possessed a sense of rectitude over procedures, clarity of communication and, not least, his own reputation. His social life was probably very limited (there being very little time left between adding up, writing letters, inspecting insanitary property, listening to councillors and travelling to London on parliamentary business); his sense of humour was of the sarcastic magisterial variety not well appreciated by those many people in public life to whom irony, even in modest doses, is threatening.

In 1846 Duncan was appointed to the new post of Medical Officer of Health for the Borough of Liverpool (population about 340,000) and began his duties on 1 January 1847, in the middle of the worst social and mortality crisis in Liverpool's history, an exogenous 'event'. The arrival of 300,000 destitute Irish and the typhus many brought with them, marked him and his office in significant ways. He survived that, and the cholera of 1849, to establish a small but effective section of the Health Department, which monitored the health of the town and provided advice and authority to those charged with improving it. Through the 1850s he perfected his system of collecting mortality data, published his annual reports, reported weekly to the Health Committee, extended his operations especially into the regulation of lodging houses, kept up his correspondence locally and with public health officials in other places, had two children, and increasingly suffered himself from periods of illness. He died in office in May 1863 at Elgin in the north of Scotland. His career had fallen neatly into two; sixteen years as a hospital doctor, physician in practice, and campaigner; sixteen years as a municipal medical officer. His young widow Catherine presented many of his books and papers to the Health Department. The letter of acknowledgement from his successor, the Irish physician William Trench, was fulsome in a way that suggests that William Henry's beatification was already under way.[10]

---

[9]   W.H. Duncan, *On the physical causes of the high rate of mortality in Liverpool* (Liverpool, 1843). Originally delivered as three lectures to the Liverpool Literary and Philosophical Society in February and March 1843. So venemous were relations in the society that, according to the Reverend Abraham Hume, Duncan 'prepared, corrected, paid for, and in most instances forwarded, i.e., addressed and sent his own paper': A. Hume, *Facts and documents illustrating both the public and private history of the Literary and Philosophical Society of Liverpool* (Liverpool, 1847), p. 6.

[10]   William Stewart Trench, MD LRCS (c. 1809–77) Medical officer of health 1863–77 in succession to Duncan. Born in Jamaica and married there in the late 1830s. Graduated MD in Edinburgh in 1831, two years after Duncan, and lived close to him in Rodney Street in the 1840s. Applied to be surgeon at the Liverpool North Dispensary in February 1841 (when he lived at 32 Great George's Street) but without success. (*Liverpool Mercury*, 19 February 1841, 57a.)

Duncan's adversaries

Given the deeply-rooted vested interests that health reformers had to confront, and the ambiguity and confusion in their own ranks, it was inevitable that a web of antagonisms would entangle attempts to introduce environmental regulation and public health administration (with attendant expenditure) into a large and factious city. Though some of Duncan's adversaries were certainly hostile to him personally, their objections were first and foremost to his function. However, his relentless and stubborn pursuit of his causes, and penchant for sarcastic comment, did little to smooth his relations with those whom circumstances placed in potential conflict with his duties as medical officer. It could be argued, therefore, that one of the criteria for judging Duncan's success is the extent to which he was able to avoid conflicts, over and above those imposed upon him by local tensions and administrative and legislative confusions beyond his control. Put another way, would the battles described below have taken the same course had the medical officer for Liverpool been another man?[11]

Opposition took four main forms. Firstly, there were those for whom the very existence of a publically-paid medical officer was anathema. Secondly, there were those whose economic interests were inevitably threatened by his activities: the owners of property and businesses likely to transgress local sanitary laws, and municipal boosters and merchants for whom the persistent identification of Liverpool with ill health was unwelcome. Calling Liverpool 'the most unhealthy town in England' was no way to make friends with those whose task was to attract visitors and traders. Thirdly, he had medical adversaries, mostly surgeons. These fraternal antagonisms were only partly a reflection of the universal party squabbles over contagionist theories. In a free market, with medicine for sale, the merits of one treatment over another could be debated in public, leaving patients to purchase treatment as they chose. During epidemics, legions of quacks, as well as qualified men, seized their moment to make reputation and money out of fear. In such circumstances the presence of official medicine with the authority of municipal government (and powerful allies in central government) was bound to cause conflict. Fourthly, the Sanatory [sic] Act of 1846, which established the public health machinery in Liverpool, contained a fundamental flaw.[12] Under the Nuisance Removal Act the Select Vestry of the *Parish* was responsible for administering medical relief and for taking preventive and ameliorative measures during epidemics, whereas the Liverpool Sanatory Act gave the responsibility for preventive measures to

---

[11]   I am grateful to Professor Christopher Hamlin for discussion on this point and for his comments on other aspects of an earlier draft of this chapter.

[12]   An Act for the Improvement of the Sewerage and Drainage, and for the Sanitary Regulation of the Borough of Liverpool: 9 and 10 Vict. cap. 127.

the Corporation of the *Borough*.[13] Thus the seeds of conflict were *built into* the legislation; the local Act clashed with the national law. Duncan had, in part, to work through a body who were not only charged with responsibilities but also with raising the money to pay for them. He therefore had to gain their co-operation either through goodwill or by going to their masters in Whitehall. Professional jealousies being what they are, he and the Health Department were to be at loggerheads with the Vestry. There were many others with whom Duncan had heated, often prolonged, exchanges of words, including William Farr on at least two occasions, but in Farr's case at least these were the result of clumsy misunderstandings by men on the same side.

All these conflicts cut across party politics in unpredictable ways. Certainly the Health Committee, as well as the whole Council, had its share of reformers keen on all health-promoting measures and (as far as the ratepaying voters would allow – which was not far) ready to pay for them. It also had 'economists' for whom public expenditure and municipal regulation were close to blasphemous. Most covered the ground between and were selective in the health measures that they would support.[14] The Health of the Town Committee, formed in about 1842, and its successor from January 1847, the Health Committee, were chaired by a succession of Tories. Not until 1852 did a Reformer occupy the chair.[15] Duncan appears to have cared little for factions or party politics; if he had strong allegiances he kept them well hidden. He was essentially a professional who regarded his expertise and professional status as an independent source of authority. His correspondence, the source of what we know about his official activities, is, unsurprisingly, discrete about his municipal employers.

Duncan was certainly not a man who went out of his way to make enemies, though once he sensed a fight was necessary he did not hesitate to go for the jugular. He was acutely aware that the commercial interests of the port needed protecting. His letters to foreign consuls, reassuring them about the state of epidemic disease, especially cholera in 1849, can be read as attempts at damage limitation.

---

[13]   Nuisances Removal and Diseases Prevention Act [1846]: 9 and 10 Vict. cap. 96. This temporary measure should not be confused with amending Act of 1848, or the subsequent Acts with same short title.

[14]   The factions and personal and family loyalties of the reformed Liverpool Council after 1835, many of whose members were from the old freemen families of the pre-reform oligarchy (and also, incidentally, members of the Select Vestry with open conflicts of interest) have yet to be uncovered. The history of municipal politics in Liverpool between the Municipal Corporations Act and the Second Reform Act of 1867 needs to be tackled. Liverpool is the one great Victorian city absent from Asa Briggs, *Victorian Cities* (Harmondsworth, 1963).

[15]   James Aspinall 1842–44, Ambrose Lace 1845–47, J.A. Tinne 1848, James Parker 1849–51 and Edward Langsdale 1852–.

Several episodes could be selected to illustrate aspects of Duncan's work and the obstacles he faced as he did battle for public health. Those selected here address three quite distinct circumstances, yet all show him working not as a medical hero but as a rather unpopular, or at best grudgingly respected, environmental manager. In the first, through the almost accidental way in which Duncan's appointment became a full-time one, we see not an enthusiastically supported and well-funded new initiative – municipal public health under medical direction – but the half-hearted appointment of a respected local medical practitioner to a job whose description was so vague that one suspects the Council was unaware what they were doing. The second episode demonstrates the the way that an epidemic can banish reason in face of self-interest and in doing so cut across otherwise well-drawn lines between progressive and reactionary forces. The third episode demonstrates the confusion of moral and medical objectives in Victorian public health, born of inadequate understandings of both epidemiology and the lives of the urban poor.

Parsimony or principle? Opposition to a full-time medical officer

Duncan's appointment was at first a part-time one to enable him to carry on his private practice. Attitudes to the new office were mixed and Duncan required support in high places to secure his base.

On 5 January 1847 a full meeting of the Council agreed that Duncan be appointed medical officer. Only James Parker, porter brewer and right-wing Tory, opposed the choice. There had been no advertisment in the newspapers as was required by the Council's standing orders for any expenditure of over £20.[16] In an obvious reference to Duncan, Parker spoke of those 'who talked more and forced themselves into notice'.[17] But he was alone: Alderman Nichol claimed that had the whole medical profession of the town been consulted there would have been an overwhelming majority for Duncan.[18] So the choice of the man was uncontroversial, indeed, probably widely approved. The real doubts were over money and the nature of the job. The salary (£300) and terms of appointment were to cause disagreement.

Edwin Chadwick had been asked to give a testimonial for Duncan. He was fulsome in his praise. Noting that he had first met him in September 1840 in the company of Dr William P. Alison, Dr Neil Arnott and Dr [Robert] Cowan in an investigation of the slums of Glasgow, Chadwick commended Duncan's

---

16   *Liverpool Chronicle*, 2 January 1847, 5. *Liverpool Journal*, 2 January 1847, 3.
17   *Liverpool Mail*, 2 January 1847, 2f.
18   *Liverpool Times*, 5 January 1847, 5. On Parker see Hugh Shimmin, *Pen and ink sketches of Liverpool councillors* (Liverpool, 1866), pp. 64–6.

evidence to the Health of Towns Commission as 'one of the most valuable pieces of service that have in their own time been rendered to [the] population' of Liverpool.[19] But this was more than a personal testimonial, it was a characteristic (and 3,350-word) memorandum on the nature of the job, which must have rankled in Liverpool Town Hall. Chadwick poured scorn upon the inadequacy of the salary and upon the evils of a part-time appointment. Claiming the premature death of an adult cost the community £325, he argued that Liverpool required three full-time medical officers of health 'at an expense of £2,200 per annum, which, if efficiently directed would be a very economical expenditure, as powerfully tending to reduce the annual charge of £18,000 for the excess of funerals alone'.[20] A third of £2,200 is close to the salary Duncan was to be given for full-time employment at the end of his first year in office. A local surgeon, Richard Reid of Bootle, had also written to a local newspaper objecting to the low salary.[21] On part-time appointments, Chadwick wrote:

> Regular private practice not only acts constantly as an inducement to the neglect of regular public duties, but often as a severe penalty for the proper performance of them. In tracing the causes of epidemics, the officer of health must at least occasionally find it in the mismanaged or neglected state of properties owned by his patients, or by persons holding local public office, persons of powerful influence, who sooner or later may exert it to his prejudice.[22]

Chadwick compared the extravagance of St George's Hall, then under construction, with the parsimony of the medical officer of health's salary, and further suggested that a statue of Dr Currie be placed in St George's Hall in testimony to earlier warnings about the sanitary state of Liverpool which were ignored.[23] Chadwick concluded in typically pugnacious style:

> Dr Duncan, after his reports, and the demonstration of their truth, can really have stood in no need of any testimonial from me; and should the considerations I have submitted be deemed too late to alter the arrangements, I would beg to present this as a personal testimonial in the way of protest against the precedent of allowing private practice on the part of an officer of health to come in conflict with his public duties.[24]

---

[19]   *Liverpool Times*, 19 January 1847, 3. A copy of the full testimonial dated 8 January 1847 was sent to the Home Secretary on 14 January and is extant: Public Record Office (hereafter PRO) HO45/1824. See also University College London (hereafter UCL), Chadwick papers, 2181/12/35 f. 65 Chadwick to Duncan 28 October 1845.

[20]   Ibid.

[21]   *Liverpool Journal*, 2 January 1847, 5; letter of 24 December 1846.

[22]   Ibid.

[23]   *Liverpool Times*, 19 January 1847, 3.

[24]   *Liverpool Journal*, 16 January 1847, 16.

The appointment drew sarcasm from *Punch* – how could a 'competent person', a 'respectable medical gentleman' be secured for £300? A doctor in private practice would find it impossible to be fully independent of local interests:

> If the Officer of Health recommended by *Mr. Punch* shall have for a patient a rich butcher, with a slaughterhouse in a populous neighbourhood; an opulent fellmonger or tallow-chandler, with a yard or manufactory in the heart of the town, he shall not hesitate from motives of interest to denounce their respective establishments as nuisances. He shall not fail to point out the insalubrity of any gasworks, similarly situated, the family of whose proprietor he may attend; and if any wealthy old lady who may be in the habit of consulting him shall infringe the Drainage Act, he shall not fail to declare the circumstances to the authorities.[25]

Despite all this advice, the Town Clerk wrote to the Home Secretary asking him to approve the appointment and stating that 'as the Officer is quite new the Council have not at present the opportunity of ascertaining the extent to which the time of the Officer will be occupied by the important public duties devolved upon him but if after the experience of a Year or so it is found that private practice is incompatible with the efficient discharge of those duties the Council will be prepared to reconsider the subject'.[26] But in his reply, Sir George Grey stated his objections to the part-time status of Duncan's appointment, suggesting in fact that he may need further assistance to complete the work even if employed full-time: he refused to confirm the appointment and the matter remained unresolved.[27] Sutherland and Chadwick had been instrumental in securing this rebuke to the Council. A month after Chadwick penned his long testimonial for Duncan, Sutherland wrote to Chadwick complaining of the part-time nature and low salary of the post. While noting that 'No better man could be appointed than Dr Duncan', and that 'It is true Duncan has accepted the office conditionally', he added that 'I am sure that one man's whole time & attention is if anything too little for such a place as Liverpool'.[28] The low salary and part-time nature of the job set a bad example

---

[25]   *Punch*, 12, 1st quarter 1847, p. 44a. This lampoon on the parsimony of the Council did not go down well in some Liverpool circles: *Liverpool Mail*, 30 January 1847 2b.

[26]   PRO HO45/1824: Town Clerk of Liverpool to Sir George Grey, 25 January 1847. It is not known why the Town Clerk waited nearly three weeks after the agreement in council to write this letter.

[27]   LivRO HC mins 1, 58ff, 15 February 1847; *Liverpool Mail*, 27 February 1847, 3a.

[28]   UCL, Chadwick papers, 1920/1, f. 2, Sutherland to Chadwick, 8 January 1847. This reference and those which follow are to the copybooks of Chadwick's own letters. The page references are to the folios within the volume.

which smaller towns would only exacerbate: 'The idea being that no competent man will act unless an adequate salary be offered'.[29]

Sutherland assured Chadwick that 'Duncan does not know that I am writing to you'.[30] Chadwick had long ago attended to the question in his letter of 8 January to the Town Clerk of Liverpool. As he told Sutherland, he had written:

> [A] very long letter of remonstrance having been asked by Dr Duncan for a testimonial. I sent in a protest. I should be glad if you could see it. I have sent to Mr Philip Holland of Manchester a copy of it. I hope it will be published in the local papers & the Medical Journals for I feel as you do upon it. I had not looked into the act until I had written the letter. I now see that the appointment is subject to the approval of the Secretary of State. I shall certainly make representations upon it.[31]

Sutherland also told Chadwick that his 'very long letter of remonstrance' had 'produced a great sensation here & I have no doubt its effect will be salutary in more ways than one'.[32] Sutherland was 'not without hopes that your remonstrance has had effect: for Dr Duncan has not yet received his appointment'.[33] Sutherland was unable to get a deputation of the Liverpool medical profession together to protest the terms of the appointment, due to a lack of unity on the question. After the letter was sent from Sir George Grey, Sutherland sent premature congratulations to Chadwick:

> I am highly gratified to learn that your remonstrance has been effectual; and that to your other services in the cause of Sanitary Reform, you had added this one, of having saved the whole movement from a great danger. I trust that there will be no such attempts again and that the precedent of interference on the part of the Secretary of State, with the doings of our Town Council, will teach the other public bodies what they may expect if they mistake their duty in a similar manner.[34]

Sutherland agreed surreptitiously to secure the publication of Grey's letter in the *Liverpool Journal*, on the following Saturday.

Yet, despite all this effort and scheming, Hamlin argues that Chadwick was ambivalent about the need for medical officers which were a last-minute addition to the Public Health Act of 1848, and that the pressure for them came from the medical profession.[35] If this applies to Duncan's case, as Hamlin

---

[29]   Ibid., f. 3.
[30]   Ibid., f. 4.
[31]   UCL, Chadwick papers, 1920/1, f. 2, Chadwick to Sutherland, 9 January 1847.
[32]   UCL, Chadwick papers, 1920/1, f. 6, Sutherland to Chadwick, 8 February 1847.
[33]   UCL, Chadwick papers, 1920/1, f. 7, Sutherland to Chadwick, 8 February 1847.
[34]   UCL, Chadwick papers, 1920/1, f. 10, Sutherland to Chadwick, 18 February 1847.
[35]   Hamlin, *Public Health and Social Justice*, pp. 255–6.

indeed suggests, then Chadwick was further down the spectrum from deviousness to dishonesty than we may have supposed.[36]

Eventually the post of medical officer became full-time almost without anyone noticing. At the last meeting of the year, the Lodging Houses Sub-committee presented its recommendations on the duties of the medical officer of health. The statement on the need for a full-time appointment could almost have been written by Duncan himself:

> it is impossible that he can, if he discharge his manifold public functions, have any spare time at his disposal for private practice, and that even if he had such spare time, he would be placed in circumstances where his private interest must necessarily conflict with his public duties. If those public duties are faithfully discharged he may probably from time to time incur the hostility of those who may have the power and be willing to exercise it of injuring him in his private professional capacity.[37]

The sub-committee went on to specify the medical officer's duties with regard to lodging-house inspection and the examination of graveyards and slaughterhouses. The concluding resolution of the report was: 'That it be recommended to the Council to appoint Dr Duncan as Medical Officer exclusively devoted to the duties of his Office. That subject to the approbation of the Secretary of State it be recommended to the Council to pay Dr Duncan a salary of £750 per Annum and that Dr Duncan be required to give up all practice'.[38] Since the Home Secretary had objected to the part-time appointment in the first place the approbation was hardly necessary.[39] It was not just patients Duncan had to give up, he also had to cease lecturing at the infirmary.[40]

Even if his personal position was regularised to his satisfaction, Duncan continued to labour without staff. By 1854 the 202 employees of the Corporation who were the responsibility of the Health Committee represented 43 per cent of the £54,583 municipal salary bill. Duncan himself had no personal staff, though by 1864 his successor had a staff of seven in addition to himself.[41] In February 1851 he famously replied to a council circular (and how

---

[36]   Professor Hamlin in private correspondence with me, September 1997, applies the general argument to the case of Duncan: 'Chadwick was highly ambivalent about the need for the post *unless it did work for him*' [my emphasis]. This leaves a puzzle, for in Hamlin's view of Chadwick's narrow concept of public health he can have had *no* expectations of Duncan.

[37]   LivRO HC mins 1, 476, 30 December 1847.

[38]   LivRO HC mins 1, 479, 30 December 1847.

[39]   But compare the way the City of London handled the employment of John Simon.

[40]   LivRO HC mins 1, 611, 20 April 1848.

[41]   *A Return ... of all the officers employed or paid by, the Corporation; with the names and salaries of their predecessors.* (Liverpool, 1854). *A Return ... of the names, occupations, and salaries of all the officers, clerks, and servants in the employ, or paid by, the Corporation*

familiar this story is) demanding a list and particulars of staff in his department:[42]

> Dear Sir,
> Your note of 1st. Inst. requesting a Return of all persons in my department paid by the Corporation to be forwarded to you by Monday morning at Ten o'clock was only delivered at my office on Monday evening at ½ past Five. I was therefore unable to comply with your request.
> The following List comprises the whole of the Officers in my Department paid by the Corporation,
> William Henry } Medical Officer }
> Duncan M.D.   } of Health   }   }£750.—.—

For many of his opponents, Duncan continued to be regarded as a mere statistics gatherer, not deserving of a full-time post at public expense. William Trench, Duncan's erstwhile neighbour and colleague, faced the same problem. As soon as he replaced Duncan in 1863 there were demands for his post to return to a part-time one. Some bodies of opinion had long memories and had never accepted that the post be full-time.[43]

Nimbyism: the case of the fever sheds

The timing of Duncan's appointment and the typhus epidemic of 1847 made Liverpool a particularly interesting testbed for relations between the nascent municipal health authorities and the older bodies that had come to administer health services, though it is a special rather than a representative case. In his first report to the Health Committee in early February 1847, Duncan gave an extraordinarily detailed account of fever cases ward by ward, even for one street, which suggest very close co-operation with the Poor Law district medical officers.[44] He issued recommendations not just to the Health Committee, but also to the Vestry, as the body responsible for sanitary measures during epidemics. In particular, he asked for additional fever wards since the fever hospital had been full for months. Legislative confusion and

---

of Liverpool ... on the 31st December, 1859, 1864, and 1869 ... (Liverpool, 1870). Both in LivRO H 352 005 COU.

[42]   LivRO MOH letter books 1, f. 421. Duncan to Shuttleworth, 4 February 1851.

[43]   *Liverpool Daily Post*, 26 May 1863 quoted in W.M. Fraser, *Duncan of Liverpool. An account of the work of Dr. W.H. Duncan Medical Officer of Health of Liverpool 1847–63* (London, 1947), p. 147.

[44]   W.H. Duncan, *Report to the Health Committee of the Borough of Liverpool, on the health of the town during the years 1847–48–49–50, and on other matters within his department* (Liverpool, 1851), pp. 5–21.

Duncan's relationship with the Poor Law Commission (via Chadwick and the General Board of Health) made him a threat to the independence of the Vestry and were to cause the fiercest conflicts of his career. At this stage, however, the parochial authority responded positively.

In early April 1847 the Vestry, prompted by Duncan, erected three fever sheds on open ground beside the workhouse on Mount Pleasant, which, as its name suggests, was an airy hill overlooking the town and in an area of fashionable residences. The district (Abercromby ward) also contained the residences of many leading physicians and surgeons and the Liverpool Medical Institution. The simple act of building three sheds, each approximately 38 by 11 metres, caused a storm of protest from residents. Long before the first patients arrived on 13 May, the new wards had caused a stir and had become a catalyst for wider action on the Irish pauper question. A powerful local lobby of the classic 'not in my backyard' variety did not want them opened at all.[45] The nearby residents of Abercromby ward were against the siting of the sheds in their area. Less than a week after construction began, complaints had reached the voluble councillor William Earle.[46] By 23 April a local surgeon, Hugh Neill, had informed the press of local alarm and a variety of objections began to emerge: the area was 'populous' and the triangular arrangement of the sheds would cause infection to spread in all states of the wind.[47] A public meeting on the 24th was followed by a deputation to the Health Committee at the Town Hall of some fifty to sixty people, including Councillor Robertson Gladstone, John Cooper, surgeon and the chairman of the deputation, Dr John Sutherland, Dr James McNaught, Hugh Neill, and James Radley, manager of the Adelphi Hotel.[48] A memorial signed by 200 people contained a comment by John Sutherland which probably captured the general mood: 'only two days ago, I was consulted by a family in the neighbourhood, who are looking out for a new house, as they will not live near the new fever wards. I would not be an alarmist, but I think the feelings of the public ought to have been consulted before so very important a step was taken.'[49] Others brought stories of those who let rooms and were facing ruin. The medical board of the workhouse was dismissive of the sheds which they claimed would, even when dry enough for use, hold only fifty-six patients each; but their main objection was that they had

---

[45]   The common informal acronym, nimby (not in my back yard) is strictly anachronistic but entirely apt.

[46]   The main objections at this stage, when the buildings were already having window frames fitted, were that the movement of sick and dead could be seen from nearby houses. *Liverpool Mercury*, 13 April 1847, 188c, 16 April 200d.

[47]   *Liverpool Mercury*, 23 April 1847, 216c; *Liverpool Mail*, 24 April 1847, 5c.

[48]   *Liverpool Mercury*, 27 April 1847, 221f.

[49]   Ibid.

not been consulted.[50] The Health Committee promised that a sub-committee would confer with Dr Duncan in the morning, an idle promise since Duncan was in London on Water Bill business. At the Select Vestry the following day a sub-committee of four members of the Health Committee arrived to discuss the sheds, so that they could be properly informed for a public meeting that evening. They got little more than vague assurances that all would be done to minimise any nuisance: 'The walls will be raised and the ventilation so managed as to prevent danger', by which they meant making holes in the floor.[51] One vestryman with a long memory remarked that no complaints had been made by local residents when cholera sheds were set up in the Haymarket in 1832. The meeting in the Phoenix Inn that evening was not reassured; it pleaded with the Vestry to hold its plans and arranged another meeting for the following week.[52] At that meeting the leading role of the medical profession was obvious. At least five physicians and eight surgeons attended, most of them living in fashionable addresses nearby.[53] The remarks of the chairman, John Cooper, are worth quoting in full:

> The Chairman referred to an anonymous letter which appeared in the *Albion* on the subject of the fever sheds, in which the author showed himself to be a non-contagionist. That had nothing, however, to do with the question. It was whether fever should be brought into such a densely populated neighbourhood as that of Mount-pleasant, to the great deterioration of property; and whether fever were contagious or otherwise, the parish authorities ought not to be allowed to ride roughshod over even the prejudices of the people.[54]

The meeting was told that Dr John Sutherland, Duncan's colleague in the local public health lobby but also a resident of the area, was in London with two local petitions against the sheds which Sutherland would present, respectively, to the Home Secretary and to the Poor Law Commissioners. He was also to see

---

[50]   Ibid. The complaint about lack of consultation was in italics in the press report.

[51]   *Liverpool Mercury*, 30 April 1847, 230e. *Liverpool Mail*, 1 May 1847, 3c. See also UCL, Chadwick papers. 1920/1, f. 15, Sutherland to Chadwick, 17 May 1847.

[52]   *Liverpool Mercury*, 30 April 1847, 230d.

[53]   This was a district full of physicians and surgeons living close to their wealthy and influential patients as well as the Medical Institution. The medical men named were a handful of the many living very close by but they do include seven who lived within 300 yards of the sheds: George Watson MD, John Sutherland MD, John McNaught, John Cooper, and John Moffatt MD were respectively at 4, 10, 20, 35 and 37 Bedford Street North; Joseph Anderson MD and John Poole at 9 and 23 Oxford Street; Hugh Neill at 115 Mount Pleasant. *Liverpool Mercury*, 4 May 1847, 236a.

[54]   *Liverpool Mercury*, 4 May 1847, 236a.

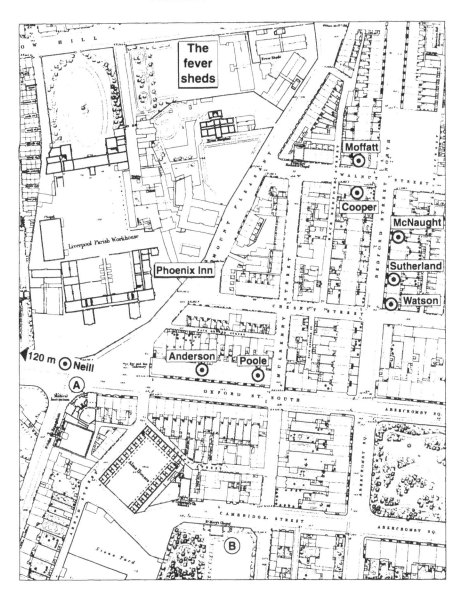

Figure 5.1: Liverpool Workhouse and the fever sheds surveyed in 1848. Part of an Ordnance Survey 'five-foot' (1:1,056) plan reproduced at 1:2,2882 (1 cm/28.8 m). Facing the workhouse wall are the modest houses of those who let lodgings, and behind them those of the professional élite. The houses of the medical men opposing the sheds are indicated. Note the Liverpool Medical Institution (A) and the parochial pauper cemetery (B) where the pauper fever facilities were buried. Original map reproduced by permission of the Trustees of the National Library of Scotland.

Lord Sandon and William Brown MP.[55] Among the recommendations contained in a letter to Sutherland from the meeting was the suggestion that the sheds be built in open country in Wavertree or Allerton. The fear was that once filled they would become permanent.

Thus a very local concern had become a *cause célèbre*. At a public meeting in the Session House, chaired by the Mayor, to 'take into consideration the best means to be adopted to relieve the ratepayers from burdens likely to be entailed upon them by the influx of Irish paupers', the matter of the fever sheds was debated. Edward Rushton, the stipendary magistrate at the centre of the whole Irish immigration question, was received with loud applause. He vigorously defended the fever sheds as 'a credit to the town of Liverpool'; he denied that they posed any threat or gave off any putrid smell.[56] In particular, he censured Neill for stirring up opposition to them. Neill had been to the Chadwick Street sheds, stood downwind of them and remarked that the smell 'resembled the odour from a steamboat overcrowded with my unfortunate countrymen'.[57] The *Mercury* saw all this as fuel for the engine of public health agitation:

THE AGITATION IS SUCCEEDING: LIVERPOOL IS TO BE PROTECTED. On the 15th of January we commenced the agitation; we have never let it subside; and now, thanks to the exertions of the Mayor and Mr. Rushton; thanks to the representations made to Government, by the Select Vestry and the Guardian Society; thanks to Lord Brougham for his speeches in the House of Lords; thanks to Mr. Surgeon Neill's suggestion of floating hospitals, in our paper; and, *above all*, thanks to Dr. Sutherland and the members of the deputation of Abercromby Ward, and our representatives in Parliament, respecting the inrush of pauperism and disease into Liverpool, the town is to be protected.[58]

Meanwhile, the Vestry stood firm. Duncan, as ever stubbornly unmoved by politics and factions, gave his support. He insisted that the Select Vestry having improved ventilation and installed water-closets at the sheds had met all

---

[55]   LivRO HC mins 1, 174–5, Duncan to W[alter] W[ren] Driffield 1 May 1847, Duncan was writing from Sheffield where he was on business concerning the Water Bill. He had met Sutherland in London the previous day. See also *Liverpool Mercury*, 4 May 1847, 236a. William Brown, the Irish-born Liverpool philanthropist was MP for South Lancashire from 1846.

[56]   *Liverpool Mercury*, 14 May 1847, 259a–d. The report on this two-hour public meeting on Wednesday 12 May is approximately 7,900 words. It gives an excellent flavour of the feeling of leading citizens on the matter, and those of Edward Rushton and William Rathbone in particular. *Liverpool Mail*, 15 May 1847, 3e–f.

[57]   *Liverpool Mercury*, 14 May 1847, 259d. The clash between Rushton and Neill was, on the surface, about whether his words were properly reported and represented. The *Mercury* took Rushton's side.

[58]   *Liverpool Mercury*, 7 May 1847, 248c.

reasonable local objections. In a letter to the Town Council's attorney, he conceded that unfounded fear prevailed but thought action would be better directed against 'those who are frightening the inhabitants out of their senses without due cause'.[59]

Writing to Edwin Chadwick a fortnight later, Sutherland was unrepentent yet saddened by the affair. His first comment was to assure Chadwick that although the fever sheds were near his house he had been reluctant to get involved: 'I have taken a part almost against my will'. Once residents found out what the buildings were for, 'they got alarmed & went quietly to remonstrate with the authorities but without success.' Sutherland showed the editor of the *Mercury* his technical proposal for ventilating the sheds, and it was urged on the Vestry by a councillor, to no avail. As alarm spread, lodgers and tenants started to leave, causing hardship to those who let their houses. Three house owners asked Sutherland to form a deputation to the Town Council from the ward: two had received notice to quit on property worth £500 and £300 a year respectively. He told them he had no fear of contagion spreading, 'but that as property was endangered I should go with them'. He described the deputation, the first of several, as a large one, but it gained no redress. Sutherland, already in London, was given powers to act for local residents. He met Sir George Grey who agreed to authorise lazaretto ships for fever cases; 'but in the mean time they have occupied the Fever Sheds and the public alarm continues'. Again Sutherland told Chadwick of his failure to persuade 'a gentleman ... who is moving his family out of the neighbourhood' that there was nothing to fear.[60] Sutherland was right in one respect, the houses on Mount Pleasant overlooking the sheds were occupied by petty tradesmen, widowers, and persons keeping lodgers.

In the same letter to Chadwick, Sutherland raised the controversial matter of the siting of fever wards in relation to open space. In his view the Vestry should have built the sheds a mile away on open corporation land where 'they might have accommodated 1000 patients & not come within a furlong or a furlong and a half of any building'. Instead, one of the sheds was 7 yards from the nearest houses 'and the people can see into that shed from their drawing room windows'.[61] Regardless of Duncan's reassurance, in a further letter to the Poor Law Commissioners, that only a 'purely imaginary' danger lay behind 'any injury to property which may arise from a groundless alarm,' the Health Committee supported the claims of the residents against the Select Vestry.[62] Still the residents persisted with further memorials to the Select Vestry and,

59   LivRO HC mins, 175. Duncan to W.W. Driffield, 1 May 1847.
60   UCL, Chadwick papers, 1920/1, f. 15, Sutherland to Chadwick, 17 May 1847.
61   Ibid.
62   LivRO HC mins 1, 181, Duncan to Assistant Secretary to the Poor Law Commissioners [W. G. Lumley], 8 May 1847.

accompanied by Sutherland, they went there one last time on 13 May.[63] In early June the matron, Mrs Todd, told the chairman of the Workhouse Committee that she thought alarm in the neighbourhood was subsiding, and commented that if only people would come into the sheds and see for themselves 'they would be convinced how little cause there was for such alarm'.[64]

This public squabbling reveals the reluctance of the wealthy to have the hospitals of the poor in their midst, while admitting the need for such hospitals in the abstract. It also shows the power they could exercise in making their protest. When a memorial was presented by those living near the Chadwick Street sheds, their worries were dismissed in more summary fashion. On this occasion, Duncan's reassurances were more acceptable to the Health Committee: 'Theory and experience alike justify me in giving this opinion in the most decided terms. No instance is on record so far as I am aware, of the contagion of Typhus Fever having been propaged [sic] under such circumstances'.[65] At least one councillor drew out the obvious implication of this contrast in the Health Committee's treatment of the residents of the two locations. At a meeting of the Town Council on 5 May, Samuel Holme, while himself urging the removal of the fever sheds from Brownlow Hill (though his firm had built them without the contract going to tender), was forced to admit that 'He was rather afraid that the remarks which had been made about the fever wards in one situation and the little that had been said about them in another, indicated an opinion that the lives of the poor were of less importance than the lives of the rich. (No, no)'.[66]

Sutherland's position was a difficult one. These were his neighbours and, while he did not share their fears, he sympathised with the consequences for their rental income. They may also have been among his private patients. They may have been among Duncan's private patients, too, in this his first year in office when his appointment was only part-time. There was also a difference of emphasis on the question of urban hospitals. The choice between urban sites, close to the homes of the sick and amenable to the control of contagion, and sites in open country, was predicated on conflicting theories of contagion and possibly the priorities of medical care and teaching. It was to recur for many years in several towns and cities.[67] On one side, reformers such as Chadwick,

---

[63]   *Liverpool Mail*, 15 May 1847, 3e–f.

[64]   *Liverpool Mercury*, 8 June 1847, 318c.

[65]   LivRO HC mins 1, 199, Duncan to the Chairman of the Health Committee [Ambrose Lace], 27 May 1847.

[66]   *Liverpool Mail*, 8 May 1847, 3e. For a report on the failure to place tenders, and opposition from one of the churchwardens, George Riding, see *Liverpool Mercury*, 6 April 1847, second edn, 182e.

[67]   I am grateful to Christopher Hamlin and Gerry Kearns for comments on this context, which merits further exploration than is possible here. R. Lambert, *Sir John Simon, 1816–1904*,

Nightingale and Sutherland were against them: 'I am a strenuous advocate of treating all *collections* of the sick in the purest air and would remove all hospitals of all kinds to a distance from towns'.[68] On the other, Simon and Duncan were in favour of them on grounds of convenience to the poor and the physical danger of moving sick people too far for treatment.[69]

This issue returned in later epidemics when the choice between home treatment, urban houses of refuge (fever hospitals) and rural hospitals would again be debated. Nothing came of a proposal from the Town Council that the Health Committee consider providing two fever hospitals for non-pauper patients although the matter was referred to Newlands for report.[70] Consequently, hospital provision fell upon the Parish, in the case of paupers, and upon the Infirmary in the case of others. Duncan was convinced of the value of hospital provision. In April, he reported that: 'During the last fortnight the proportionate mortality among the Fever patients treated at their own Dwellings has been on a rough estimate nearly double of that among the patients treated in the Hospitals, a fact which shows the propriety of providing ample Hospital accommodation for the treatment of such cases'.[71] The many fevered sick turned away from the fever wards represented a missed opportunity for cure, but also remained as a threat to others since, in Duncan's view, they could 'communicate the contagion to the other inmates of their rooms and cellars'.[72] His attempts to get the Select Vestry to provide adequate hospital accommodation can not have been helped by the opprobrium heaped upon the Brownlow Hill sheds by members of his own profession.

Duncan must have been especially irked by the role of his friend Sutherland. In early May the Vestry wrote to the Home Secretary requesting military tents to serve as emergency wards. Sir George Grey offered to open the government stores at Chester Castle to supply the Select Vestry with two large tents suitable for convalescing fever patients.[73] Despite an intervention by the Mayor, and an instruction by Grey to his secretary to write to the Mayor 'to say that I have requested the Bd. of Ordnance to direct their storekeeper at Chester Cassle [*sic*] to deliver on the requisition of the Mayor any spare tents which may be

---

and English Social Administration (London, 1963), pp. 479–83 for Nightingale versus Simon on the siting of St Thomas's Hospital.

[68] UCL, Chadwick papers, 1920/1, f. 16, Sutherland to Chadwick, 17 May 1847.

[69] Lambert, *Sir John Simon*, pp. 479–83.

[70] LivRO HC mins 1, 73, 3 March 1847; 86, 8 March 1847; 91, 15 March 1847.

[71] LivRO HC mins 1, 140, Duncan to the chairman of the Health Committee [Ambrose Lace], 10 April 1847.

[72] LivRO HC mins 1, 157, Duncan to the chairman of the Health Committee [Ambrose Lace], 17 April 1847.

[73] *Hansard* 92, House of Commons, 7 May 1847, c.526.

required', it does not seem that the tents ever arrived.[74] This may be because the Select Vestry proposed to pitch them in front of the workhouse near the much-disputed sheds and, given Sutherland's influence with Grey through Chadwick, this might explain Grey's conditional offer only of tents 'if places could be found outside the town where they could be fixed'.[75] The fever sheds served their purpose, but Duncan had been somewhat thwarted by one he regarded as his closest ally.

The lodging house question and the Reverend Cecil Wray

The second view of Duncan in battle comes from his determination to regulate lodging houses, which, in common with most Victorian health reformers, and Chadwick in particular, he regarded as a crucial source of infection and means of rapid dissemination of disease among the vast number of footloose casual poor.[76] The issue is a particularly interesting one in that it illustrates how far environmental and social regulation could be pushed by local authorities ostensibly in the interests of public health, but in reality revealing that characteristic urge towards social control of the dangerous classes, medicant lodgers and all those living in irregular domestic arrangements. The characteristic emphasis on the moral and social evils of unregulated lodgings, followed by their filthy and unventilated condition, was reflected in the journal of the Liverpool Health of Towns Association: 'the only way of avoiding them in future is to place all lodging houses under strict control; a step which is contemplated by the Liverpool Sanitary Improvement Act'.[77] Lodging houses had long been identified as a public health issue but the question has been largely explored by historians in the context of London and the two Shaftsbury Acts of 1851, the one to regulate existing houses, John Simon's 'ragged dormitories', the other to empower authorities to build model lodging houses.[78]

---

[74]   PRO HO45/1816, Item 4, Letter of George Hall Lawrence, Mayor of Liverpool, to Sir George Grey, 13 May 1847. At an emergency Vestry meeting on 18 May it was stated that the tents would soon be arriving and that they would probably be placed in front of the workhouse. *Liverpool Mail*, 22 May 1847 3a.

[75]   *Hansard* 92, House of Commons, 7 May 1847, c.526.

[76]   M.W. Flinn (ed.), *Report on the Sanitary Condition of the Labouring Population of Great Britain by Edwin Chadwick 1842* (Edinburgh, 1965), pp. 411–21.

[77]   J. Sutherland (ed.), *The Liverpool Health of Towns Advocate*, part 2 (London and Liverpool, 1847), 151–2. First published as issue no. 16, 1 December 1846.

[78]   E. Gauldie, *Cruel Habitations, A History of Working-class Housing 1780–1918* (London, 1974), pp. 240–50. Simon is quoted on p. 241. A.S. Wohl, *The Eternal Slum. Housing and Social Policy in Victorian London* (London, 1977), pp. 74–8. For a local enquiry into lodging houses in the 1830s see H. Marland, *Medicine and Society in Wakefield and Huddersfield 1780–1870* (Cambridge, 1987), p. 344. Engels, drawing on J.P. Kay's survey of

Glasgow and Liverpool were well ahead of London and anticipated Shaftesbury's Bills on this issue. The effectiveness of the Liverpool system of registration is shown by a comparison with London. Although the provisions of the 1846 Liverpool Act incorporated in the City of London Sewers Act of 1848, the City and most other parts of London conspicuously failed to emulate Liverpool both in regulating lodging houses and prosecuting keepers.[79] The matter occupied Duncan a great deal in the late 1850s and dominates the third volume of his correspondence as he wrote letter after letter attending to the details of the registration and inspection of individual lodging houses.

The unskilled migrant made up a particularly large part of the town's population and it is likely that footloose lodgers in common lodging houses (staying anything from a day or two to several weeks or months, as distinct from the arrangement of lodging families found in all Victorian cities) were more prevalent than in most cities.[80] Whatever the reason, the 1846 Sanitary Act included a single, but effective, section to deal with lodging houses, taken virtually word for word from section 20 of the Calton Burgh Police Act of 1840. Its place in the Liverpool Act was probably the work of Chadwick and Duncan, though it is puzzling that the further powers in the Calton Act concerning infectious diseases in lodging houses were not copied in Liverpool.[81]

In summary, the Act stipulated that all lodging houses (excluding public houses or inns licensed by magistrates) be registered and their keepers named in a register book; that their capacity be fixed by the Council or its Health Committee; that in every room there be posted prominently a notice of the number of lodgers allowed and the regulations regarding health, cleanliness and ventilation; that access be given to officials at all times for the purpose of inspection, inquiry, or disinfecting; and that fines not exceeding 40 shillings

---

condition in Manchester in 1831 suggested that 5,000 to 7,000 people in the township lived in lodging houses or 3.5 to 5 per cent of the population: F. Engels, *The Condition of the Working Class in England* (Oxford, 1958), p. 77. See also Flinn (ed.), *Report on the Sanitary Condition of the Labouring Population*, p. 24.

[79] V. Zoond, *Housing Legislation in England 1851–1867, with Special Reference to London* (unpublished MA thesis, University of London, 1932), pp. 62–89 but especially p. 66 and pp. 79–80. I am grateful to Gerry Kearns for drawing my attention to this thesis.

[80] I know of no study of the Victorian lodging house which quantifies their presence in different cities. Nor is it known how long most lodgers stayed in such houses. Lyon Playfair, quoting Duncan's *Physical Condition*, provided the nearest thing to a statistical overview in the Second Report of the Commission on the Health of Large Towns and Populous Districts. Liverpool lodging houses had, on average, 6.4 beds and compared with other Lancashire towns were far better supplied with sanitary facilities. Parliamentary Papers 1845 [610], xviii. 325–7.

[81] 9 and 10 Vict. cap. 127, section 125. The Calton Burgh Police Act, April 1840: 3 Vict. cap. 28, sections 20–22. Duncan's excursion with Chadwick to the slums of Glasgow in September 1840 suggests that he had long known of the Calton regulations.

could be imposed on keepers failing to comply. The purpose of these provisions, which remained unaltered in Duncan's time, was stated with admirable clarity in the preamble (which also defines the nature of lodging in such places as 'for the night or other short periods'), to prevent overcrowding and the consequent communication of infection. No other purposes are stated or hinted at.[82]

In June 1859 the Medical officer of health assumed full responsibility for the process of regulation and his letters (over 200 of them are wholly or partly concerned with the issue) throw light on the day-to-day work of the inspectors.[83] Duncan frequently complained of overcrowded lodging houses and regularly ordered that infected persons or infected bedding be removed by the police.[84] The first lodging house by-laws came into operation in August 1848.[85] About fifteen police officers were appointed as inspectors of lodging houses and instructed to visit suspected unregistered houses at night and if necessary lay informations against their keepers. They were also to visit registered houses to ensure they were not exceeding the number of lodgers for which they were registered. By 15 December 1849, after sixteen and a half months of operation, 311 persons had been charged with not registering and 133 registered keepers with overcrowding. Such cases went before the stipendary magistrate, Edward Rushton, who, Duncan informed the General Board of Health, interpreted clause 125 'to apply exclusively to houses receiving *nightly* lodgers'.[86] Although the number of charges of overcrowding was high, '30 per cent of the entire number of registered houses', Duncan took the view that most of these were in the early months of operation, and that once the Council's serious intent became clear, most lodging house keepers quickly fell into line.[87] Magistrates almost invariably imposed the full fine and many

---

[82]   Under section 203, dealing with by-laws and regulations, the Council was empowered to make regulations for registering lodging houses, and for keeping them clean and 'in a wholesome condition'.

[83]   LivRO MOH letter books 2, f. 468. Duncan to Rathbone 6 July 1859. W. H. Duncan, *Report on the health of Liverpool during the year 1860* (Liverpool, 1861), p. 16.

[84]   Three crucial memos describe the by-laws and their operation, and the Medical Officer's duties in this area. The clearest statement of the operation of the Liverpool system comes from the first Inspector of Nuisances, Thomas Fresh, *Report to the Health Committee of the Town Council of the Borough of Liverpool, comprising a detail of the sanitary operations in the Nuisance Department, from 1st January, to 31st March, 1851* (Liverpool, 1851), pp. 29–39. A sharper assessment of how the system of registration and inspection worked in practice can be pieced together from fragmented records. The registers themselves do not appear to have survived, though the minutes of the Lodging Houses Sub-committee have.

[85]   LivRO MOH letter books 1, f. 295, Duncan to General Board of Health (hereafter GBH), 15 December 1849.

[86]   LivRO MOH letter books 1, f. 297, Duncan to GBH, 15 December 1849.

[87]   LivRO MOH letter books 1, f. 297, Duncan to GBH, 15 December 1849.

defaulters were gaoled.[88] Duncan estimated that 90 per cent of registered keepers were Irish. In January 1861 there were nearly 700 registered houses in Liverpool and some unregistered; in 1860, the first year of his new system of regulation now transferred from the police to the Health Committee, there were over 35,000 inspections.[89] This was a huge addition to his prodigious workload, yet he prepared carefully, for example taking advice from Henry Letheby, Simon's successor as medical officer for London, on inspection and the possibility of separating the sexes, and was as *dirigiste* as ever.[90] Duncan had a contemptuous view of lodging house keepers generally. When new offices were being planned for the Health Department, he wrote to James Newlands: 'I hope [mine] is one which will be easily found by very stupid people, a number of whom (in the shape of Lodging house Keepers etc.) call on me daily'.[91]

Lodging houses were thus bound to lead to trouble and were soon the subject of characteristic recrimination by letter, with Theodore Rathbone (brother of William Rathbone V and a prolix agitator on lodging houses), with Captain Elgee, the Chief Constable of Lancashire, and with Cecil Wray. Rathbone, whose repeated claim was that Liverpool was full of unregistered lodging houses, bombarded the medical officer with pedantry for some months, becoming increasingly personal in his attacks, so that Duncan, after penning over 4,000 words to him, lost patience and terminated the correspondence.[92] Rathbone's name carried some weight and he encouraged Elgee to complain of Duncan to the Mayor and the press. For his pains, the Chief Constable received his own epistolary bloody nose.[93] Duncan's spat with the Reverend Cecil Wray, a senior Anglican clergyman in the town who almost died of typhus fever in 1847, was more significant. It was to be his last fight, and from his sixteen letters on the affair we gain a clear impression of Duncan's character and of the precise nature of the regulatory mind at work. Wray's letters to the

---

[88]   LivRO MOH letter books 1, f. 297a, Duncan to GBH, 15 December 1849. The local newspapers bear out Duncan's view, though by 1860 there were complaints in the Health Committee that the magistrates were being soft on lodging-house keepers: *Liverpool Mercury*, 4 May 1860, 7e.

[89]   W.H. Duncan, *Report on the health of Liverpool during the year 1860* (Liverpool, 1861), pp. 16–17.

[90]   LivRO MOH letter books 3, f. 33. Duncan to Letheby, 14 November 1859.

[91]   LivRO MOH letter books 3, f. 85. Duncan to Newlands, 24 February 1860.

[92]   LivRO MOH letter books 3, ff. 46–7. Duncan to Rathbone, 2 December 1859. *Liverpool Mercury*, 5 October 1859, 3f–g; 14 October 1859 7a–b; 19 October 1859 3f–h; 18 November 1859 7b.

[93]   LivRO MOH letter books 3, ff. 46–47. Duncan to Elgee, 16, 22 and 24 October 1860.

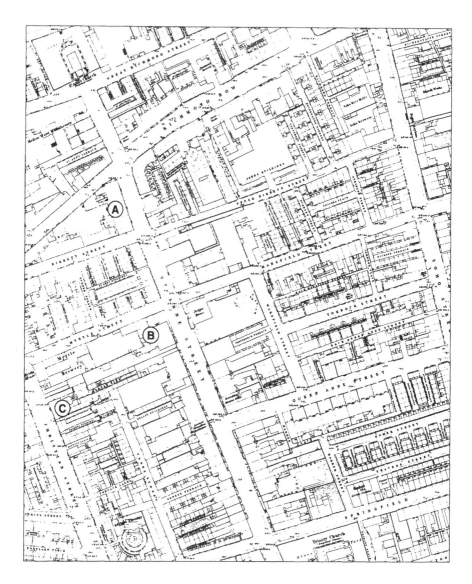

Figure 5.2: Cecil Wray's model lodging houses. Part of an Ordnance Survey 'five-foot' (1:1,056) plan surveyed in 1848 and reproduced here at 1:2,882 (1 cm/28.8 m). St Anne Street was surrounded by crowded court housing more than a decade before Wray established his houses.(A) 107 St Anne Street.(B) 20 Holly Street (renamed from Myrtle Street about 1860).(C) 80 Christian Street, established as a model lodging house about 1870. Original map reproduced by permission of the Trustees of the National Library of Scotland.

Health Committee carry a genuine sense of grievance and a great deal of plausible argument.[94]

Wray, the incumbent of St Martin in the Fields, a prominent church in a none the less poor district of Liverpool, seems to have had an interest in model lodging houses from at least the early 1850s.[95] By 1864 he had five such establishments, including one at 107 St Anne Street and another close by at 20 Holly Street, both large houses of the 1790s in a once fashionable quarter now full of tradesmen and labourers.[96] In early February 1859, at precisely the time when he began to take personal command of lodging-house regulation, Duncan arranged to meet Wray at his model house in Great Oxford Street, off Scotland Road, with James Pope, the district medical officer. The stated purpose was to allow Pope to point out defects 'likely to promote disease', but in the matter of sanitary inspection Duncan needed no second opinion – as he was to tell Wray two years later, 'in the matter of eyesight I consider *myself* competent'. Pope failed to attend, but was informed by Duncan that the house had 'no ventilation whatever': unsurprisingly, in February, lodgers were in the habit of papering over ventilation holes.[97] In March 1860 Duncan informed Wray that the keeper of one of his lodging houses was to be prosecuted for overcrowding.[98]

The scale of Wray's new model house in St Anne Street, twenty rooms for 107 lodgers, can be gauged from Duncan's letter to him the following November, in which details of the capacity of every room are set out and stringent requirements for washing and ventilation are stipulated. It is not hard to imagine Wray rankling at Duncan's prescriptions: 'the space allowed to each lodger in the Rooms Nos 16 and 22 is rather less than I think desirable in a *Model* Lodging house'.[99] In late January 1861 the house was still not registered and Duncan, painstaking as ever yet trying to be flexible (in a comradely tone which probably irritated Wray) insisted that the regulations be fulfilled to the letter. The rooms had to be numbered permanently: 'we adopt the London mode of marking the number with a scribe on the inside of the door, but you

---

[94]   LivRO Lodging House Sub-committee minutes 17 February 1862, 17 March 1862 and 19 May 1862.

[95]   Duncan agreed to meet him at a model lodging house in Great Oxford Street, off Scotland Road and near his church of St Martin in the Fields on 8 September 1852. The lodging house was his personal concern rather than a parish institution. LivRO MOH letter books 1, f. 536. Duncan to Wray, 4 September 1852.

[96]   He may have had others, for *Gore's Liverpool Directory* for 1864 gives five premises under a single entry 'Model Lodging Houses', including those in Great Oxford Street and Limekiln Lane near his church of St Martin's also listed in 1859.

[97]   LivRO MOH letter books 2, ff. 449–52. Duncan to Wray, 9 February 1859 and to Pope, 9 and 15 February 1859. Pope failed to attend.

[98]   LivRO MOH letter books 3, f. 86. Duncan to Wray, 2 March 1860.

[99]   LivRO MOH letter books 3, f. 137. Duncan to Wray, 28 November 1860.

would probably wish to paint them, or adopt some other plan'.[100] Wray had obviously indicated that he wanted the St Anne Street house to be registered under the 'Common Lodging Houses Act' which suggests that proprietors had a choice between the Local Act and the General Act.[101]

Duncan was not a man to offer special favours, even to prominent local clergy. The intense regulation finally caused Wray to lock horns with him in late January 1862 in a series of claims and counter-claims: Duncan wrote eight letters in two weeks and Wray at least four. Clearly, Wray had accused Duncan of simply wishing to cause annoyance through officiousness. Duncan's testy but patient replies, pointing out complaints from lodgers and inspectors – the state of vermin-infested blankets, unchanged sheets, failure to post notices, blocked up windows, and so forth – reveal simultaneously his dogged character and the extraordinary attention to detail. The regulations alone would have been insufficient to effect improvement; the character of the medical officer was crucial, and general lessons cannot necessarily be drawn from the Liverpool case. Even so, that leaves the question of whether the rigorous system of inspection really did have health benefits for poor lodgers or whether it merely provided an opportunity for officials to exercise control and be seen to do so.

Wray claimed that his lodging houses had been subjected to an unnecessary 'repetition and severity of inspection' while other unfit houses went undetected.[102] Duncan, probably suspecting a cleric expecting special treatment, clearly objected to the way Wray advertised his premises as 'model' lodging houses: 'I have no objection whatever to a public investigation, which can very easily be procured, and the result of which would probably satisfy even yourself that at the *time of inspection* that house was by no means entitled to the appellation of a "Model" Lodging house'.[103] As the two sides dug in, Wray made wider and wider charges of suppressed facts and falsehoods. Even with only Duncan's side of the correspondence, the suspicion remains that Wray had some justification for his rage at bureaucratic oppression; it is doubtful whether the lodging house inspectors used the same patient logic as Duncan. But Duncan returned to the law time and again, and was clever in taking a superior moral position:

---

[100]   LivRO MOH letter books 3, f. 156. Duncan to Wray, 26 January 1861. In April 1861 it was still not a lodging house, being occupied by a Welsh joiner and his family: PRO RG9/2694/50v.

[101]   14 and 15 Vict. c.28 [1851] Duncan was officially made responsible for registration under the Common Lodging Houses Acts of 1851 and 1853 in November 1860: LivRO HC mins 6, 601, 9 November 1860.

[102]   LivRO MOH letter books 3, f. 264. Duncan to Wray, 31 January 1861.

[103]   LivRO MOH letter books 3, f. 263. Duncan to Wray, 29 January 1859.

The rule then is that every Lodging house should undergo a day inspection once a week on an average and a night inspection about once a fortnight. From this rule your lodging houses have been exempted – an exemption for which I have been blamed and which I now believe cannot be wholly justified. The fact is that your houses have *never* been visited at night, and never even during the day, except on the complaint of a lodger, and on such occasions the result has proved the necessity of the visit.[104]

Wray had made a serious error in taking Duncan on. Even to imply that he was not even-handed in the exercise of his duty was to invite a devastating reply.

When I complain of this statement as a charge (not against myself but against those whose duty it is to report unregistered houses) you say it does not amount to a *charge at all*, and where I ask you to give me the address of *any one* of the unregistered houses to which you refer you are unable to do so but say you will try to find some out! In common fairness I must say, the finding out should have preceded the positive assertion. Such a charge, for charge it is, should not have been made on the mere chance of being able to 'hunt out' facts in its support.[105]

Time and again he corrected Wray as to precisely what he had written, and he entrapped Wray into sending him a list of houses which he claimed were unmolested by registration and inspection, all of which turned out to be outside the provisions of the Act, including a brothel.[106] He even came close to accusing Wray of fraud and deception:

I think it right to let you know that all of the houses (with one exception) in your list, were found to have been visited on Saturday last by men, who by means – it is said – of false representation, induced the keepers in several instances to promise to provide accommodation for one, or for two, lodgers; with the view – it is supposed – of reporting them as liable to registration. The story told by the man or men in nearly all the seventeen cases was that they wished to secure lodgings for some stone masons who were to arrive in Liverpool on that Monday. In several cases the parties were put to much trouble & inconvenience in consequence, & one poor woman complains that she went to the expense of 4/- on the faith of the promise that two lodgers would be with her on Monday evening. This ~~had~~ woman as well as others in the list – had never at any time received lodgers.

104 LivRO MOH letter books 3, f. 264. Duncan to Wray, 31 January 1859.
105 LivRO MOH letter books 3, f. 267. Duncan to Wray, 1 February 1859.
106 LivRO MOH letter books 3, f. 270. Duncan to Wray, 6 February 1862.

I need not say that none of the stonemasons have yet made their appearance.[107]

As usual, Duncan covered his back well by getting support from the Health Committee and the full Council; he sent copies of all his correspondence with Wray to Charles Bowring, chairman of the Lodging Houses Sub-committee, to which Wray's own letters of complaint had been referred by the Health Committee.[108] A very full report on the whole business, especially the allegations of perjury by inspectors, was approved on 17 March 1862. Wray, seeing it in late April, after some absence from Liverpool, returned to the fight after taking advice from 'some friends'. Duncan began again to demolish his arguments. Clearly wishing to end the business, Wray wrote to Duncan assuring him that he imputed no ill motives and signalling a declaration of peace. He wrote to Thomas Dover, chairman of the Health Committee, on the same lines referring to 'the Report of Dr Duncan'. The next day he received a reprimand: Duncan denied that it was his report. Technically it was not, but he clearly wrote it and it is not to his credit that he failed to drop the matter.[109] Within a year, Duncan was dead. Wray, his contemporary, died in 1878. In 1881, 107 St Anne Street and 20 Holly Street were still called 'model' lodging houses and on census night gave shelter to 273 adult male lodgers from a wide variety of occupations, including a surgeon.[110]

The battles in perspective

What emerges from all these battles (and those in which Duncan took a back seat, such as the water question which split parties, caused councillors to lose seats, and became the great *cause célèbre* of the 1850s) is a sense of relentless bickering. The Council and its Health Committee achieved almost nothing through consent, let alone enthusiastic consent. The powerful bureaucratic influence of the medical officer was often resented; he was viewed by more than a few as a busybody with little to do except collect figures and interfere in private property. On the other hand, the Borough Engineer, James Newlands, was held in high regard; the benefits of his efforts were there for all to see (if sewers and water pipes can be said to be visible) and his work had obvious appeal to those keen on promoting civic improvement through order and public

---

[107]   Ibid., 270–71.

[108]   LivRO MOH letter books 3, f. 269. Duncan to Wray, 4 February 1862. LivRO Lodging Houses Sub-committee mins 17 February 1862.

[109]   LivRO Lodging Houses Sub-committee mins 19 May 1862. LivRO MOH letter books 3, f. 269. Duncan to Wray, 13 May and 21 June 1862.

[110]   PRO RG11/3631/54–57 and 76–78v.

works, and especially to developers in the suburbs where the infrastructure was being provided at public expense.[111]

The essential first step in assessing Duncan's contribution to public health is to distinguish between his diagnosis and his remedy. The second is to distinguish between the short-term and long-term results of his work. As a diagnostician he was brilliant – painstaking, precise and perceptive. In all their elaborated forms in modern studies as well as contemporary reports, Duncan's statistics have been the almost exclusive basis for the analysis of patterns of mortality in Liverpool.[112] His statistical methods were both sophisticated and effective, given the state of the data, the state of statistical science in 1840, and the public appreciation of statistics.[113] There can be little argument that he fulfilled admirably his primary duty, to monitor disease and to report to the Corporation. Despite his early difficulties with the registrars and in some cases district medical officers of the Vestry, he perfected a geographic information system of considerable sensitivity. He also managed to do this with the fraternal co-operation of the parochial medical officers in a way that seems to have eluded John Simon in London.[114]

In these selected episodes I have used the model of a man with battles to fight, and thus human enemies as well as enemies in nature and circumstances, as a means of presenting his career and those aspects of public health in which he was prominent. It is an appealing metaphor. Because of the way Duncan (a well-decorated general but no Field Marshal) – and his compatriots in the 1840s – identified the enemy and determined on the battle plan, the presentation and priorities of Victorian public health became fairly fixed for decades to come. If Duncan's wish was to demonstrate to public satisfaction that his was the best way to fight sickness and the causes of sickness, the proof

---

[111]   C. Hamlin, 'James Newlands and the bounds of public health', *Trans. Historic Society Lancashire and Cheshire*, 143 (1994), 117–39. In February 1849, a member of the Health Committee spoke of 'the perseverance, industry, and talent of our very clever borough engineer' *Liverpool Mercury*, 13 February 1849, 99. Newlands, whose salary from 1853 was a third more than the medical officer's, received a huge civic funeral in 1871: *'In Memoriam;' or, Funeral Records of Liverpool Celebrities* (Liverpool, 1876), pp. 183–7. See also S. Sheard, 'James Newlands and William Henry Duncan: a partnership in public health', *Trans. Lancashire and Cheshire Antiquarian Society*, 87 (1991), 102–21.

[112]   Either via his own reports or his evidence to Parliamentary enquiries. J.H. Treble, 'Liverpool working-class housing, 1801–1851' in S.D. Chapman (ed.), *The History of Working-class Housing* (Newton Abbot, 1971), pp. 165–220; R. Dennis, *English Industrial Cities of the Nineteenth Century. A Social Geography* (Cambridge, 1984), pp. 56–63.

[113]   P. Laxton and G. Kearns, 'Statistics and the management of public health: the methods of W.H. Duncan M.D. 1805–1863'. Paper given to the Social Science History Association Annual Conference, Baltimore, Maryland, November 1993.

[114]   Simon failed to get co-operation from parish surgeons in London partly because he seems not to have had the character or persistence to work with these humble medical toilers. Lambert, *Sir John Simon*, pp. 115–16.

certainly did not come in his own lifetime. Liverpool was as sickly and dangerous for the working class in the late 1860s as it had been in the early 1840s.[115] In his own career he demonstrated an iron belief in his philosophy and procedures, a fact that may well have contributed most to his reputation among his fellow professionals, but it is for historians to judge the long-term legacy against the short-term achievement, and to continue to question whether, as in warfare, the victorious generals are the best people to write its history.

Acknowledgements

This paper is associated with a project by the author and Dr Gerry Kearns (Jesus College, Cambridge), supported by a grant from the Wellcome Trust for the History of Medicine, to publish Duncan's correspondence. I am especially grateful to Gerry Kearns, to our Research Assistant Mrs Joy Campbell and to Helen Grant for typing the letters. Professor Chris Hamlin's comments have been invaluable even where I have failed to rise to the challenge.

---

[115]   The average annual crude death rates (unweighted) for Liverpool and West Derby registration districts for 1842–46 were 33.8 and 25.4 per thousand respectively. For 1864–68 they were 40.9 and 28.9. These differences cannot be explained by poor death registration in the early of the two quinquennia.

6

Town Hall and Whitehall: sanitary intelligence in Liverpool, 1840–63

Gerry Kearns

The Public Health Act of 1848 and the Local Act of 1846

In the public health reports of the 1840s, Liverpool was often taken to exemplify the evils of the unregulated, insanitary city. Much of this evidence about Liverpool came from local experts, particularly Samuel Holme and William Henry Duncan. As the chapter by Paul Laxton explains, Duncan was a local doctor who went on to become the first British full-time Medical Officer of Health in Liverpool in 1847. Prior to his appointment he had established himself as the obvious candidate for the new post by virtue of his studies of sanitary conditions in the town. Duncan described the cellar and court dwellings of Liverpool to three successive sanitary inquiries. To Slaney's inquiry of 1840, he promised that cleaning the dwellings of the poor would easily pay for itself in reduced pressure upon the poor rates.[1] For Chadwick's 1842 report he rehearsed the miasmatic theory of fever and the importance of drainage and sewerage, scavenging and cleansing.[2] In 1843, Duncan wrote a pamphlet reviewing the failures of the recent [1842] Local Act. A slightly abbreviated version was then published in the evidence of the 1844 Buccleuch Commission.[3] The conclusions reached by the public health activists presenting these reports, and in particular by Chadwick, was that without housing regulations and sanitary engineering, large towns and cities were deadly to the poor and dangerous to the rich. The failure of local authorities to act upon this fact was attributed to their ignorance, obduracy and laziness. The only

---

[1]   British Parliamentary Papers [PP]1840 (384) xi, 277, 'Report from the Select Committee on the health of towns', 141–51.

[2]   PP 1842 (HL-) xxvii, 1, 'Local reports on the sanitary condition of the labouring population of England', 282–94.

[3]   W.H. Duncan, *On the physical causes of the high rate of mortality in Liverpool, read before the Literary and Philosophical Society in February and March, 1843* (Liverpool, 1843); abridged in PP 1844 [572] xvii, 1, 'First report of the Commissioners appointed for inquiring into the state of large towns and populous districts. Appendix', 12–32.

conceived solution was to bring these facts more efficiently to their attention through some system of centralised reporting and publication and to enforce their adherence to certain minimum standards of good practice through compulsory regulations. Thus, the Bishop of London was acting as a good disciple of Chadwick when he inserted into the 1848 Public Health Act a clause which triggered the compulsory application of the Act to any place showing a significant increase in the number of deaths due to epidemic disease.[4] Yet using the extremity of such as Liverpool to promote compulsory legislation for the whole country was not acceptable to all. When, in discussing the abortive Health of Towns Bill of 1847, William Brown urged its necessity on the grounds that 'In Liverpool ... they strongly felt the want of proper sanitary regulations', Richard Spooner replied that Liverpool's special circumstances justified a special and not a general measure.[5] Certainly, those considering the advisability of passing a Public Health Act were invited to contemplate the woes of Liverpool as sufficient justification.

In Liverpool, the lessons were equally clear if somewhat different. It was obvious that Duncan's pamphlet and its national prominence had gained the town a certain notoriety: 'showing that Liverpool was then the lowest as regarded longevity of any town in the kingdom'.[6] Duncan himself spoke to the Liverpool Health of Towns Association of the 'stigma ... justly attached to the town of being the most unhealthy in the kingdom'.[7] Local opinion was also keenly aware of the contrast between, on one hand, the wealth of many of Liverpool's merchants and the opulence of such buildings as St George's Hall, then under construction, and, on the other, the desperate poverty and short life-expectancy of the town's poor. This implied painful criticism of both the efficiency and the humanity of the local authorities. Beyond this, a commercial centre contemplated with some anxiety the effect on trade of being presented as a place dangerous to visit, work in or live in. But there were many in Liverpool who simply refused to accept the picture painted by Duncan and retailed by the parliamentary reports. Duncan had to answer local pamphlets which simply denied the evidence of the Registrar-General's returns, arguing that Liverpool

---

[4]   *Hansard* 100 House of Lords, 27 July 1848, c.894; ibid., House of Commons, 7 August 1848, c.1174. This idea of relying upon a deterioration in the death rate was altered in the Commons to the apparently more workable criterion of a crude death rate of twenty-three per thousand.

[5]   William Brown, merchant with interests in Liverpool. Born in Ireland. In 1847 he was a Liberal pro-free trade MP for South Lancashire. He was later to become a major benefactor of the city of Liverpool, providing it with an art gallery and library. Richard Spooner, Protectionist Conservative MP for Birmingham. *Hansard* 93 House of Commons, 1 July 1847, cc.1094–5.

[6]   *Liverpool Chronicle*, 27 May 1854, 7.

[7]   *Liverpool Mail*, 27 February 1847, 5b.

was, indeed, exceptionally healthy apart from the anomaly of a community of the Irish poor who inflated all the mortality returns. This mortality, the critics believed, did not reflect upon conditions in Liverpool but instead represented mortality exported from Ireland itself.[8]

One of the points which clearly impressed the local authorities of Liverpool, as it did those of other places, was that sanitary legislation was inevitable. The reforming Whig ministry brought in on the tornado of the Reform Act of 1832 had dealt a root-and-branch reform to the Poor Law and to local government. Nor were conservative interests safe with the Tories. They, after all, had repealed the Corn Laws, freed Catholics and Nonconformists from many civil disabilities and, indeed, had passed the Reform Act itself. Far better, it seemed to many, to secure a Local Act which would secure the legitimate aims of the Public Health Act without subjecting the town to the sort of intrusive central control exemplified in the much-disliked new Poor Law. Beyond this, there were yet others who believed new legislation unlikely and that these promoters of a Local Bill were certainly persons expecting to gain thereby in some personal capacity, as officers of the new authority perhaps. Nor were some impressed with the quality of intelligence derived from parliamentary reports. A local Liberal newspaper exasperated with the 1844 Royal Commission under the Duke of Buccleuch, accused it of doing no more than regurgitating the findings of Duncan's pamphlet without taking the country any further toward a solution:

> 700 pages in folio to prove what no man in his sense ever thought of questioning, viz., that the filthy state of our great towns, the incommodious plans of their buildings and streets, and other arrangements, are the main causes of the frightful mortality which decimates the poor ... [W]e expected from this volume something more than the unpretending pamphlet of Dr. Duncan had already communicated; but we regret to say that no recommendations have been made by the Commissioners which specifically refer to us. Indeed, the report itself only occupies eight pages ... without advising anything.[9]

Yet, in Holme's evidence to the 1842 inquiry, there was just such a blueprint and something like it became the basis for the Local Act.[10]

---

[8]   W.H. Duncan, *Letter to John P. Halton, Esq., in reply to his strictures on 'The physical causes of the high rates of mortality in Liverpool'* (Liverpool, 1844). Liverpool Medical Institution, Pamphlets vol. 23, no.7.

[9]   *Liverpool Mercury*, 2 August 1844, 256b.

[10]   PP 1844 [572] xvii,1, 'First report of the Commissioners appointed for inquiring into the state of large towns and populous districts. Appendix', Replies from Samuel Holmes, 185–95; 9 and 10 Vic. c.127 [Liverpool Improvement Act No. 20] 'An Act for the improvement of

The Local Act drew upon the emphasis on the regulation of buildings characteristic of Normanby's unsuccessful bill of 1844, and upon the local experience of the failures of Liverpool's Local Act of 1842 as described by Duncan in his pamphlet.[11] As Paul Laxton shows, the Local Act also drew upon the lodging house regulations of Glasgow of which Duncan and several others had direct knowledge; Duncan, indeed, had accompanied William Pulteney Alison when Chadwick and Neil Arnott had been shown around the slums of Glasgow during the preparation of the famous Sanitary Report of 1842: as Chadwick recalled a few years after in a letter to Duncan, 'so early, so important an ally on the great question of sanitary improvement. I shall always remember your perambulation with Dr. Arnott, Dr. Alison and myself of the wynds of Glasgow'.[12] And the experiences of places such as Glasgow continued to be of interest to the sanitary officers of Liverpool. In June of 1854, for example, James Newlands, the Borough Engineer, made a report on the paving system of Glasgow.[13] In other words, the translation of local intelligence through central government was not directly relevant to the formulation of the Local Act. It was, however, indirectly necessary in that the shameful prospect of the loss of local control animated many supporters of the new measure. In terms of principles, the package defined as the sanitary idea had to be taken as a whole if local measures were to help Liverpool avoid the compulsory measures which seemed to be in the offing.

Principles and techniques of sanitary reform

To understand the roles and relations of local and central government in sanitary reform, I want to distinguish, as in Figure 6.1, between principles and techniques. The principles of sanitary reform are the abstract ideas which are universally agreed. By contrast, the techniques of sanitary reform are the instruments chosen to ensure that the goals of sanitary reform are achieved. We can identify three government functions where centre and locality came together. These are the functions of intelligence, legislation and enforcement. Intelligence denotes all those means whereby information was gathered and analysed, and conclusions published. Legislation covers both Public, or

---

the sewerage and drainage, and for the sanitary regulation of the Borough of Liverpool', June 1846.

[11]   5 and 6 Vic. c.44 [Liverpool Improvement Act No. 15] 'An Act for the promotion of the health of the inhabitants of, and better regulation of the buildings in, the Borough of Liverpool', June 1842.

[12]   University College London Manuscripts Room [UCL], Chadwick papers 2181/12, f. 65, Chadwick to Duncan, 28 October 1845.

[13]   *Liverpool Mercury*, 23 June 1854, supplement, 15.

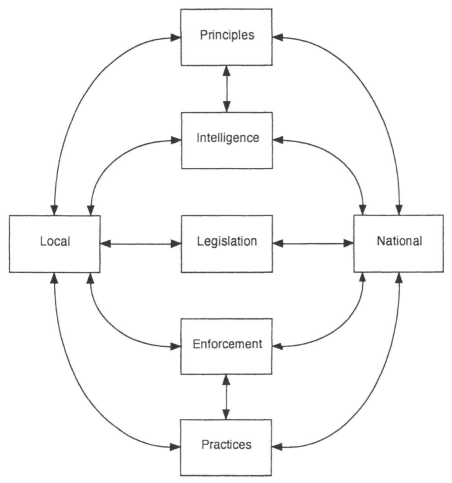

*Figure 6.1: The relations between central and local government
in the field of sanitary reform*

general, Acts of Parliament and Local Acts which are those applying to one place only, in this case Liverpool. Enforcement, self-evidently, refers to all those measures taken to ensure that the law is followed.

Here attention will be directed to the first of these three functions and consider the central–local politics of sanitary intelligence. It is important to distinguish between three aspects of sanitary intelligence: public health reports, the detection of national epidemics and the monitoring of sanitary progress. The relations between central and local administration provide occasions for co-operation, conflict and compromise. Attempting to untangle some of these relations, in the field of sanitary intelligence, I have chosen to distinguish in a rather crude fashion between the views of central government, both Whitehall and Parliament, and the reactions in Liverpool, although in many cases we might speak of the view from Liverpool and the reactions in London. I have also drawn a rough and ready division between the prevailing, or official, view and the claims of those who contested it in either central or local administration. Figure 6.2 summarises these relations for the three facets of sanitary intelligence mentioned already. For example, in the case of sanitary reports, the official view was that Liverpool could be taken as an exemplar of the problems of insanitary cities. In Parliament and before Select Committees, there were others who argued that, on the contrary, Liverpool was a city sweet and unexceptional in its filth, sickness or mortality. In Liverpool, many accepted the official view and joined in the attacks on the failures of local institutions. Yet in Liverpool, too, there were those who could see no sickness, feel no suffering and smell no filth. Three examples of 'intelligence' in public health activities will be examined in turn which relate broadly to Parliament, Whitehall and Liverpool opinion. The first is the place of Liverpool in the public health campaigns which led up to the passing of the 1848 Public Health Act, the second the place of Liverpool in epidemic intelligence, and the third is how the need for further sanitary reform was monitored and debated. In each case the view from Whitehall, the reactions in Liverpool, and the national and local opposition to the prevalent views and reactions, will be described.

These distinctions between principles and techniques and between London and the provinces have been central to debates over the nature and evolution of government and administration in this period. There are some, the fabled Whiggish historians of old, who have seen enlightenment residing in Westminster or Whitehall and who treat national legislation as attempts, at first strident, to bring enlightened modern practice to backward peripheral regions with their provincial cities and narrow world-view. This was, of course, the self-image of many of the state bureaucrats who devised and implemented the legislation, and where their biographies form the core of institutional histories of social policy, those histories can see little but central drive and local

Intelligence

	The official view	Reactions in Liverpool	
Reports	Liverpool taken as exemplar of insanitary cities	Liverpool stigmatised as notorious	Prevalent
	Exemplary nature contested	Notoriety contested	Opposition
Epidemics	Liverpool as early warning of national epidemics	Liverpool in danger	Prevalent
	Epidemic contested	Danger contested	Opposition
Monitoring	Liverpool shows need for futher national legislation	Liverpool is much improved, needs only minor changes	Prevalent
	Liverpool irrelevant as source of lessons	Public Acts take no account of local conditions	Opposition

Figure 6.2: Sanitary intelligence and the politics of central–local relations

resistance. For example, writing of the Local Government Board in the 1870s, H.J. Dyos described all the proud provincial towns who had spurned Chadwick's directives in the 1850s coming back like lost sheep for direction in the less ideological 1870s.[14] Nanny knew best, at least in technical matters. On the other hand, some such as Royston Lambert describe a central government having to abandon all ideological pretensions in favour of an incremental, pragmatic adjustment of policy in line with the technical lessons learned from the local failures of earlier central policies.[15] Christine Bellamy sees this less heated ideological climate as itself a matter of principle. She describes two models of central–local relations: the one based on central expert direction and the other more a partnership dominated by negotiation and a respect for local autonomy.[16] All three of these share a view of government growth in which the failures of the ideological 1840s and 1850s are retrieved in the more pragmatic 1860s and 1870s. Against this, we need to set the emphasis of Judith Hart upon a deeply entrenched opposition to reform which needed to be displaced

---

[14]   H.J. Dyos, 'Greater and Greater London: metropolis and provinces in the nineteenth- and twentieth-centuries', in D. Cannadine and D. Reeder (eds), *Exploring the Urban Past: Essays in Urban History by H.J. Dyos* (Cambridge, 1982), pp. 37–58.

[15]   R.J. Lambert, 'Central and local relations in mid-Victorian England: the Local Government Act Office, 1853–71', *Victorian Studies*, 6 (1962), 121–50.

[16]   C. Bellamy, *Administering Central–Local Relations, 1871–1919: The Local Government Board in its Fiscal and Cultural Context* (Manchester, 1988).

ideologically before merely practical questions could be broached.[17] We need also to recall Samuel Finer's documentation of the myriad institutional innovations of the Benthamites, in particular Chadwick, and the framework those institutions provided in the longer battle to get the social policy innovations implemented.[18]

What has perhaps been missing from many of these accounts has been a recognition of the interplay between central and local administration during which both principles and techniques were innovated, developed and tested. What follows is a preliminary attempt to assess these interactions.

Intelligence of epidemics

Central government was acutely aware of the place of Liverpool in the diffusion of epidemic disease into England. Port cities such as Newcastle, Glasgow and Liverpool had been the early sites of cholera in 1831–32 and they also featured among those places with the largest concentrations of truly vulnerable poor people. Here, if anywhere, epidemic disease was likely to strike first. Reports of fever or of cholera had central government despatching nervous letters to Liverpool seeking confirmation or denial. This was a very important part of Duncan's job.

When, in December 1846, the Select Vestry petitioned central government for controls on the immigration of Irish paupers into Liverpool and for some relief from the burden the starving Irish were placing upon the poor rates, the Home Office remained unmoved.[19] Yet the suggestion of Augustus Campbell, the chair of the Select Vestry, in his covering letter enclosing the petition, that 'fevers of a typhoid character have already appeared' had Sir George Grey writing immediately to the Mayor for confirmation. Duncan, Medical Officer of Health for the Borough from the following month of January, was instructed to respond. This he did in a detailed report which set the form and tone for many subsequent reports. His aim was to use the averages of comparable weeks in previous years to determine whether the sickness and mortality currently experienced were exceptional or not. He contacted the surgeons at the charitable dispensaries, the district medical officers of the Poor Law authorities and the Registrars of births and deaths. His findings were unequivocal. A fever epidemic was not yet afoot but its inevitable, terrible scourge was not far off:

---

[17]   J.T. Hart, 'Nineteenth-century social reform: a Tory interpretation of history', *Past and Present*, 31 (1965), 38–61.

[18]   S.E. Finer, 'The transmission of Benthamite ideas 1820–50', in G. Sutherland (ed.), *Studies in the Growth of Nineteenth-Century Government* (London, 1972), pp. 11–32.

[19]   PP 1847 [764] 1, 1, 'Memorial of the Select Vestry of the Parish of Liverpool to the Home Secretary' [dated 24 December 1846], 46.

'Should the present state of things continue and the destitute Irish still flock into the town as they have hitherto done, there can be little doubt that what we now see is only the commencement of the most severe and desolating Epidemic which has visited Liverpool for the last ten years'.[20]

All through the spring and summer of 1847, Duncan continued to send despairing reports from the eye of the storm. Yet the problem in 1847 was seen, essentially, as a problem of destitution for the Poor Law authorities. The government did not invoke its powers under the 1832 Cholera Act. It did not declare an epidemic and thus issue regulations covering quarantine and much besides through the Privy Council. On 21 September 1848, the Privy Council did just that because of the appearance of cholera in Hamburg and its likely early translation to Newcastle or some other east-coast ports.[21] The passage of the 1848 Nuisances Removal and Diseases Prevention Act at the end of August soon changed all that.[22] The new Act had been marched through Parliament at breakneck speed in order to meet the demands of this anticipated epidemic of cholera. It took the management of the epidemic away from the contagionist Privy Council and placed it with the anticontagionist General Board of Health, shifting the public health emphasis from sick bodies towards unhealthy places.[23] The cholera, in contrast to the fever, was not expected to confine itself to the Irish paupers but, following the precedent of 1832, it was anticipated that it would reach most towns and cities and would number the comfortably-off, and not just the poor, among its victims. In sanitary terms, it was a national question in a way that few understood the famine and its associated fever to be. Yet, unlike the Privy Council regulations, the new powers of the General Board of Health could only be invoked once cholera was already certified to be present in the country. As such, the General Board was more than anxious to learn if cholera was indeed present in any of its likely early haunts, of which Liverpool was one. Yet it was Newcastle that first gave the General Board of Health the confirmation it needed and on 28 September, one week after the announcement by the Privy Council, the Board invoked its own powers under the epidemic regulations of the Nuisances Removal and Diseases Prevention Act.[24]

---

[20]   Liverpool Record Office [LivRO] Minutes of the Health Committee, [HC mins] 1, 156, 15 Feb 1847; letter of 9 February 1847, Duncan to William Shuttleworth, Town Clerk.

[21]   *Liverpool Mercury*, 22 September 1848, 614.

[22]   11 and 12 Vic. c.96, 'An Act to renew and amend an Act of the tenth year of Her present Majesty, for the more speedy removal of certain Nuisances, and the prevention of contagious and epidemic Diseases'; First Reading, House of Commons, 7 August 1848; Royal Assent, 4 September 1848.

[23]   G. Kearns, 'Zivilis and hygaeia: urban public health during the epidemiologic transition' in R. Lawton (ed.), *The Rise and Fall of Great Cities* (London, 1989), pp. 96–124.

[24]   S.E. Finer, *The Life and Times of Sir Edwin Chadwick* (London, 1952), p. 339.

In 1853, again, the General Board of Health prodded Liverpool for early reports of cholera cases. Once again, it was Newcastle which allowed the General Board of Health to deploy the powers under an amended Nuisances Removal and Diseases Prevention Act. The regulations were invoked for Newcastle on 15 September and for the country as a whole on the 20th.[25] Yet on this occasion, Liverpool could perhaps have offered the General Board the excuse it sought. Duncan was on leave during all of September and in his absence his inefficient deputy, Dr Cameron, noted cholera cases among German emigrants early in the month and among the Irish by the middle of the month.[26] No report was made to the General Board of Health until Duncan sent one on 10 October. It was not until 9 September of the following year that Duncan reported cholera to be running much higher than the levels associated with ordinary English cholera and diarrhoea. Only in such circumstances would he declare the disease to be epidemic.

Duncan was aware of the heavy responsibility which lay upon him in declaring a disease such as cholera to be epidemic in Liverpool. It would immediately affect shipping visiting countries which imposed quarantine on vessels from places where epidemics prevailed.[27] At one point, when cholera was intermittently rather than epidemically present, Duncan informed the Health Committee that he had omitted the details concerning the location of cholera cases for fear of exciting alarm.[28] In 1848, Duncan ensured that the announcement of the earliest cholera cases was made by a joint committee of the Health Committee of the Town Council and the Medical Relief Committee of the Select Vestry.[29] In 1853 and 1854, no such unanimity was achieved and almost to the bitter end, the Select Vestry refused to acknowledge the presence of the epidemic disease and thus of any obligations falling upon them thereby. Cholera had been present in Liverpool discontinuously since December of 1848 but it was not until two weeks after Duncan had declared it to be epidemic that the Select Vestry could be induced to act at all: 'I regret to say that it was not until the 23d. September, when the epidemic attained its maximum, that the [Medical Relief] Committee were induced to adopt measures which although still not in all respects satisfactory, are more in accordance with the severity of

---

[25]   *Liverpool Journal*, 17 September 1853, 5; *Liverpool Albion*, 26 September 1853, 9.

[26]   *Liverpool Mail*, 3 September 1853. LivRO Medical Officer of Health Letter Books, Volume 2, 4 May 1853 to 16 July 1859 [MOH letter books 2], ff. 15–23; f. 20. Duncan to the Secretary of the General Board of Health [GBH], 8 November 1853.

[27]   As James Tryer reported to his fellow Health Committee members in the immediate aftermath of cholera being declared present in the town in December 1848. *Liverpool Mercury*, 29 December 1848, 832.

[28]   *Liverpool Mercury*, 12 May 1854, supplement, 15.

[29]   *Liverpool Mercury*, 12 December 1848, 793.

the case'.[30] To justify their inactivity, the chairman of the Select Vestry's Medical Relief Committee, Edward Bradley, repeatedly challenged Duncan's claim that there was excessive cholera and even questioned the accuracy of Duncan's returns. Upon checking the figures, Duncan found that Bradley had relied on the figures for deaths given by the registrar of each subdistrict and had omitted from his calculations those deaths which had occurred in the Select Vestry's own workhouse. Duncan was touchy on the subject because his credibility rested upon the reliability of his figures and he bemoaned the Select Vestry's having made 'a statement calculated to shake the confidence of the Public in my accuracy'.[31]

Given the economic significance of his statements about epidemic disease, Duncan strained to ensure that he provided accurate figures and a reliable interpretation. Declaring an epidemic is a political act rather than merely a medical fact. Duncan drew upon two criteria in addressing this issue. First, as someone concerned with the local epidemic atmosphere, he largely confined his attention to residents with cholera rather than to visitors or strangers who might appear with the disease upon them. Second, in line with his view of epidemics as altogether exceptional he used comparisons between years to show clear departures from earlier conditions.[32] He did this with some care, omitting from his calculations those diseases where reporting was spasmodic and infrequent rather than continuous and weekly: namely, accidents and acts of violence, often subject to coroners' inquests and 'so irregularly registered that they would prevent any fair comparison being made of the mortality of one week with another'.[33]

In the case of epidemic reporting, then, we see a clear interaction between principles and practices. The principles governing Duncan's epidemic reporting were commercial as well as medical. Nor was this inherent conflict of principles considered improper. Complaining of a committee created by the National Association for the Promotion of Social Science, John Sutherland regretted: 'All doctors you will observe, & all London doctors & the people are to report on a purely commercial matter, namely Quarantine. There is not a Liverpool man on it & not a single merchant'.[34] This treatment of quarantine as

---

[30]   LivRO MOH letter books 2, f. 250. Duncan to the Secretary of the GBH, 3 October 1854.

[31]   LivRO MOH letter books 2, f. 280. Duncan to Charles Hart, Vestry Clerk, 18 October 1854.

[32]   See P. Laxton and G. Kearns, 'Statistics and the management of public health: the methods of W.H. Duncan M.D., 1805–1863', paper given to the Social Science History Association Annual Conference, Baltimore, Maryland, November 1993.

[33]   LivRO MOH letter books 2, f. 277. Duncan to Hart, 15 October 1854.

[34]   Nightingale Papers, British Library [BL], Add. MSS., 45,751, f. 126. Sutherland to Florence Nightingale, September [?] 1859.

medically useless but commercially significant was common also to John Simon's evidence on the matter to the Royal Sanitary Commission of 1869: 'we have quarantine because if we did not keep up the show of the quarantine system other countries would quarantine us'.[35] Duncan's practice was to report the presence of epidemics only when a comparison of weekly mortalities from certain classes of disease showed the current week to be much worse than in previous years. This was his own interpretation of what it meant to speak of normal English cholera, or summer diarrhoea, passing over to something more severe, the epidemic Asiatic cholera. By focusing on exceptional mortality, Duncan guarded against crying wolf too often and also thereby both harming the trade of the port and devaluing his own credibility. He hoped in this way to acquire the authority to call the local authorities to arms against the epidemic threats he did describe. In announcing epidemics, Duncan served the intelligence needs of his local authority before those of national government. He was happy to report each and every case that showed the symptoms of Asiatic cholera but he would not be drawn into using the charged term, 'epidemic', until almost the last available moment. With its epidemic powers, the General Board of Health had a quite different agenda.

Monitoring public health measures

How were the effects of sanitary interventions evaluated? To answer that question we need to examine the use made of central and local statistics of sickness and mortality. The rates of mortality reported by the Registrar-General continued to be the main barometer of sanitary success throughout this period. The quarterly and annual reports of the Registrar-General were accompanied by interpretative essays which were scoured for any local references. These reports were also quarried by the General Board of Health in order to illustrate its own publications. In his third quarterly report of 1847, covering the height of the 1847 fever epidemic and published that November, the Registrar-General observed as follows that:

> Liverpool, created in haste by commerce – by men too intent on immediate gain – reared without any very tender regard for flesh and blood, and flourishing, while her working population was rotting in cellars, has been severely taught the lesson that a portion of the population – whether in cellars or on distant shores – cannot suffer without involving the whole community in calamity.[36]

---

[35]   PP 1868–69 [4218], 1, 'First Report of the Royal Sanitary Commission', 103, q.1863.

[36]   *Liverpool Mail*, 6 November 1847, 4a–b. The other quotations in this paragraph come from the same article.

Local opinion was quick to contest the interpretation of Liverpool's elevated mortality: 'Such fine writing may do for old women who have given up embroidery and taken to statistics, the rage and folly of the day, but it is out of place in what should be a grave report of facts as the basement of sound reasoning'. The argument in this, the Tory *Liverpool Mail*, was that conditions in Liverpool reflected not the wishes of the local authorities or the commercial classes but the poverty of so many of the town's inhabitants and the continued arrival of the 'scum of Ireland' attracted by the 'prodigality of our benevolence'. Indeed, the paper went on to say that Liverpool needed less and not more medical attention, being, in fact, 'over-doctored and over-quacked' and presently 'pestered with sanatory practitioners'. It was the *Mail*'s contention that even the Registrar-General's own 'miserably defective' statistics showed the longevity of the native inhabitants of Liverpool to be as good as in any other town. The people of the town 'are not the creators but the victims – not the nurserymen of infectious fever, but the sufferers from an inundation of wretched, starved, and diseased beggars from Ireland'.

This sort of blustery rejection of the interpretation placed on central statistics would probably not move William Farr at the General Register Office. Duncan's own response to such remarks shifted over time. At first, he would willingly accept that objective measures proved the insalubrity of the town but he would also insist that credit be given for the efforts then under way. Addressing the annual meeting of the Liverpool Health of Towns Association in February 1847, he commented as follows:

> If the stigma have justly attached to the town of being the most unhealthy in the kingdom, it is pleasing to be able to point to the exertions which are now being made by the authorities to remove that stigma, and proper that the fact should be recorded that Liverpool, as it was the first town in the kingdom to set the example of establishing baths and washhouses for the use of the poor, so it has been the first to apply for and to obtain a special sanatory enactment, and to recognise the principle that it is the duty of the municipal authorities to watch over the health and comfort of the poorest inhabitants.[37]

When Farr included this section on Liverpool in the summary *annual* report for 1847, the criticism was somewhat moderated. The jibe about the commercial classes of Liverpool having little 'regard for flesh and blood' was deleted and a footnote was added giving the Council, at least, some credit: 'The local authorities have appointed an able Health Officer, and have adopted other

---

[37]   *Liverpool Mail*, 27 February 1847, 5b.

measures, which will probably improve the health of this important commercial town.'[38]

Over time, however, Duncan questioned not only the interpretations but also the statistical methods of many central statisticians. Two examples show this very directly. In 1853, with cholera apparently imminent, the General Board of Health wrote to the local authorities at Liverpool urging them to take measures in anticipation of the disease: after all, it reasoned, Liverpool's high rate of mortality of 48 per thousand showed it to be desperately in need of some preventive measures. Preventive measures fell to the lot of the Health Committee and Duncan was asked to respond to the General Board of Health. In fact, he castigated it for falling into the 'serious error' of taking the deaths for the Borough of Liverpool and dividing them by the population of the half of the Borough which fell within the Parish and thus within the registration district of Liverpool. In fact, he told the Health Committee, the rate of mortality in the Borough of Liverpool was then 28 per thousand and had shown significant improvement over the seven years under the Local Act.[39]

In 1858, Edward Greenhow published a report for the Medical Officer to the Privy Council, the successor to the General Board of Health, in which he surveyed the current public health challenges. In it, he took Ely as an example of a well-regulated town which had shown a detectable reduction in its rate of mortality after efficient sanitary engineering. Liverpool was held up as a town having yet a long way to go. This report enraged Duncan. First, Greenhow had presented the mortality of only the Parish of Liverpool and thus had excluded the healthier outlying but contiguous suburbs included within the Borough, the unit for which the Health Committee had responsibility and the unit which corresponded more adequately with the functioning town as a whole. Yet this inner part of Liverpool was compared to whole towns, or villages, such as Ely. Second, the idea that Ely and Liverpool could ever have similar mortalities represented a ridiculous expectation according to Duncan. Whereas Greenhow, and Chadwick and Farr before him, took all mortality above the 'healthy' standard as being preventible, Duncan did not. He believed that the different circumstances of different places argued for the application of a range of healthy standards. To some extent, those he dubbed the 'sanitary censors' in London had some inkling of this, for they did not adopt the mortality level of the healthiest rural districts as an appropriate target for towns and cities.[40] Instead, they turned to the level of mortality already achieved by the best

---

[38]   *Tenth Annual Report of the Registrar-General of Births, Deaths, and Marriages in England* (London, 1852) [Report for 1847], xxiii.

[39]   LivRO MOH letter books 2, f. 97. Duncan to the secretary of the GBH, 28 November 1853.

[40]   LivRO Medical Officer of Health Letter Books, Volume 3, 26 July 1859 to 20 April 1863 [MOH letter books 3], f. 303. Duncan to Philip Holland, 7 May 1862.

towns, all small ones. Alongside the qualitative difference that they already recognised between town and country, Duncan wanted them to consider the further environmental leap which separated the market town from the gargantuan slums of cities of immigrants. After all, in the East End of London, the central statisticians had one such area on their own doorstep. Far better, he argued, to compare Irish north Liverpool with such as Whitechapel than to cast about for such as fresh and tiny Ely as a realistic measuring stick with which to beat the Health Committee.

When the 1859 meeting of the National Association for the Promotion of Social Science was held in Bradford, it received several papers on the conditions at Liverpool. Indeed, the previous annual meeting had been held in Liverpool and a sub-committee of the Public Health branch of the Association had been set up in order to prepare a report on the town for the Bradford meeting. Newlands, McGowen and several others, all gave papers. Duncan was present and took part in the discussions following these papers, as he had at the previous meeting in Liverpool. The main point of discussion was what the Liverpool sanitarians saw as the misleading and malignant way that central government besmirched the efforts of the local authorities at Liverpool. Farr felt the full brunt of the anger of those he termed 'the Liverpool squadron'.[41] But it was Greenhow and not Farr who had confused Borough with Parish, and Greenhow was not at Bradford. Following the Bradford meeting, in correspondence with Philip Holland, a sanitary reformer from Manchester but employed by the Burials department of the Home Office in London, Duncan went further and accused Greenhow of implying that it was Duncan who had confused Parish with Borough in claiming a decline from the higher mortality in the former to the lower mortality in the latter. For Duncan, this was 'too serious' a charge to be 'whispered in corners'. Duncan had 'corrected' Greenhow at the Liverpool meeting, the Bradford meeting and in his annual report of 1858. Even Holland had complained that Liverpool had 'only!' managed to eliminate one-fifth of its cesspools in the five years since the Corporation had received powers to deal with the matter: 'Verily some people have a large digestion'.[42] In sending copies of some of his annual reports to one interested party, Duncan drew his own conclusions:

> You will see that Liverpool has not had justice done to her. The men in authory. [sic] – in London – are theorists, and don't look at the practical or practicable side of the question. But I can safely say that no one who knew Liverpool 15 years ago and sees it now could do otherwise than congratulate us on what has been done.[43]

[41] Nightingale Papers, BL, Add. MSS., 45,751, f.140d. Farr to Sutherland, 30 Oct 1859.
[42] LivRO MOH letter books 3, ff. 48–9. Duncan to Holland, 2 December 1859.
[43] LivRO MOH letter books 3, f. 116. Duncan to Thomas Saddler, 3 October 1860.

In exasperation, Duncan appealed to Holland:

> If you will consent to compare the mortality of Liverpool with that of the
> east end of London, I will make no objection, but in the gloomy pictures
> which you Sanitary Censors take such delight in drawing of the town to
> whose example you allow so much, I have no recollection that you are in
> the habit of comparing Liverpool with districts of an analogous
> character, that would be obviously unfair! A little pleasantly situated
> county town or big village, like Ely, answers the purpose much better![44]

Duncan was anxious to give Chadwick some illustrations of the
effectiveness of Liverpool's sanitary efforts and he explored the possibility of
comparing fever sickness rates in streets which had and those which had not
seen improvements in drainage. He was unable to get satisfactory details on the
progress of drainage from Newlands at this time. He had more success with a
comparison of fever sickness rates between regulated and unregulated lodging
houses, but while this information found its way into the publications of Henry
Rumsey, it did not find a prominent place in those of the General Board of
Health or of the Medical Officer to the Privy Council.[45] This sickness reporting
was a fragile achievement requiring the unpaid assistance of the local Poor Law
doctors, or district medical officers. In the early years of his tenure, Duncan
made great efforts to institute a continuous system of reporting and was
certainly successful during epidemics, but the practice lapsed in the 1850s,
much to Duncan's disappointment:

> Some of the District Medical Officers occasionally report cases of Fever
> to me, occurring in their districts; but I get no systematic return, which in
> former years I often suggested as being likely to be of great public
> advantage. It has been once or twice commenced, but has always died
> prematurely.[46]

The Select Vestry was nervous about the use Duncan might make of 'their'
data, being well aware that Duncan might well use it to recall them to their
medical obligations.[47] Simon faced similar difficulties in the City of London
and was able only to consult for himself the sickness registers of the Poor Law

---

[44]   LivRO MOH letter books 3, ff. 303–4. Duncan to Holland, 7 May 1862.

[45]   See Henry Wyldbore Rumsey, *Essays on State Medicine* (London, 1856).

[46]   LivRO MOH letter books 3, f. 120. Duncan to Robert Gee, 10 October 1860.

[47]   The local registrars were appointed and paid for by the local Poor Law guardians and
were not under the sole control of the Registrar-General in London. Three sets of people might
claim some ownership over this data: the district registrars themselves who expected to be paid
if they undertook any clerical copying duties, the Registrar-General who felt able to instruct the
registrars in their local responsibilities, and the Select Vestry itself which, having paid for the
collection, thought itself justified to determine access to these data.

medical officers; no return was made to him.[48] The failure to establish any such national system of sickness reporting was a serious weakness in the national system of sanitary intelligence. Both Farr and Chadwick recognised and deplored this shortcoming.[49]

In terms of both principles and practices, there is a clear divergence between Duncan and the central statisticians. In terms of practices, Duncan did not accept that all mortality above the healthy town standard was removable from larger urban areas. He thought instead that narrower comparisons should be taken and he referred Liverpool's experience to that of Manchester, and north Liverpool's to the East End of London. Second, he was concerned more with trends than with absolute differences. He ascribed any fall in zymotic mortality to the public health efforts of the Health Committee. In doing this, he excluded epidemic years and tried to compare 'normal' years with each other. In the third place, Duncan was acutely aware of the shortcomings of the central statistics and supplemented their mortality information with the sickness data he gathered from Poor Law medical officers and Dispensary surgeons. Finally, he was alert to the lazy manner in which some in Whitehall could confuse Parish with Borough and show no awareness of the urban realities behind the statistical boxes. In this, he was part of a critical commentary upon central statistics whose most distinguished practitioner was Henry Rumsey. Yet, whereas Rumsey's harsh words were aimed even at Farr, Duncan was more exercised by those at the General Board of Health and the Privy Council who used Farr's work with a good deal less care than displayed by the compiler of abstracts himself.

There are differences of principle behind these dry statistical techniques. Chadwick and later Simon saw their problem as browbeating belligerent, lazy authorities into facing up to their sanitary responsibilities. As such, a single sanitary standard had the merit of being everywhere applicable. It also had the merit of being measurable for all places; very few collected sickness statistics of the quality and comprehensiveness characteristic of Duncan's. Very often in the national reports, local detail was used merely to illustrate general arguments and not to derive them. The sanitary idea was established in theory and no amount of local detail could drag them away from the notion that urban mortality resulted from removable sources of miasma. Evidence on local improvements only served to show that removal was both practical and effective. Their main aim was to compare the costs of sanitary works with the economic value of lives saved. There was not a suggestion that it might cost more to save lives in one place or another, or that sanitary difficulties might

---

[48] R. Lambert, *Sir John Simon, 1816–1904, and English Social Administration* (London, 1963), pp. 113–17.

[49] Finer, *Chadwick*, p. 155.

prove more intractable in one place than another. If Liverpool failed to bring its mortality down to the level of Ely, then, it was failing its citizens and the local authorities deserved to be exposed. Shame and self-interest might then lead them to follow more diligently in the footsteps of the East Anglian market town.

Duncan's approach was rather different. The Town Council had already started its march to healthier pastures when it reformed its local government and appointed Duncan and Newlands. Furthermore, they had spent large sums of money on draining, paving, sewering and water. Duncan had appealed to self-interest and shame in the campaign leading up the passing of the Local Act. Now, the task was rather different. He needed to encourage the Town Council if he were to see it make further efforts. He felt it could best be done by appealing to their pride. The Local Act had been passed with a view to maintaining the independence of the town and Duncan sought to persuade them that the success of the Local Act offered the best continuing protection of it. If the national authorities continued to decry the efforts of the Health Committee, then the economy party on the Town Council might be emboldened to scale back its extensive operations. Indeed, after Duncan's death, something like this was immediately attempted, with an unsuccessful attempt to have the post of Medical Officer of Health revert to part-time status.[50]

Conclusion

The politics of central–local relations in the question of sanitary intelligence reveals some conflicting views of the purposes and interpretation of information. In broad terms, at the time when the dominant local effort was going into squeezing a sanitary measure out of the Town Council and then defending it in committee at Whitehall, there might indeed appear to be a real convergence between the centre and the provinces. In both cases, the reformers, such as Chadwick on one hand and Duncan on the other, aimed to establish against both national and local sceptics the dire condition of Liverpool and yet its immediate improvability. Once Duncan had been appointed, his allegiance to his local masters brought new political and economic interests into play. Now, he had to maintain his local credibility by showing that sanitary intelligence was not incompatible with commercial activity. In this, he was aided by his genuine dissatisfaction, shared by many, with the effectiveness of quarantine or the need for it to be imposed on ships from Liverpool. If the anti-contagionist ideas were correct, then, epidemics were due to local conditions

---

[50]   W.M. Frazer, *Duncan of Liverpool: An Account of the Work of Dr. W.H. Duncan, Medical Officer of Health of Liverpool, 1847–63* (London, 1947), p. 147.

and not to the importation of sick people from overseas. Duncan modified his views somewhat over time, coming to see cholera as contagious in certain circumstances.[51] Chadwick and Sutherland did not, and Simon did so only to a limited degree. Yet the circumstances of contagious spread, according to Duncan, related to the handling of the dead and their linen and clothes. Neither of these directly concerned mercantile commerce. For the merchants of Liverpool, quarantining of their ships abroad followed directly upon the heels of any declaration that there was an epidemic in Liverpool. The consequences for the General Board of Health were quite different. The members of the Board had no wish to introduce a quarantine themselves, yet they could only invoke their epidemic powers when a national epidemic had been declared and thus when British ships were going to be quarantined elsewhere. There was thus an ironic divergence between the interests of the centre and the localities when it came to announcing an epidemic.

This division widened again over the question of the monitoring of sanitary progress. Here the central statisticians were, in part, the prisoners of their own techniques and sources. They had no comprehensive sickness data, only comprehensive mortality data. They were also held captive by their understanding of what preventible mortality was, and adopted a very simplistic ecological model of mortality in which there were but three categories: rural, good towns and bad towns. As Simon Szreter has shown, the sanitarians at the General Register Office defended stoutly this ecological model for the remainder of the century.[52] Duncan joined with other provincial figures such as Rumsey in calling for a more sophisticated approach to mortality analysis. Again, though, Duncan was also pulled away from the interests of the central statisticians by the new local allegiances, which followed from being in the employ of the Town Council. He thought he could point to a clear mortality benefit following from the great expenditure on sanitary engineering. Through a combination of inept analysis and inappropriate comparisons, the 'statistical censors' in Whitehall would offer his councillors in the Town Hall no such comfort.

To see sanitary reform as driven either by principle or pragmatism alone is to be misled. It is also naïve to place one, usually principle, at the centre, and the other, usually pragmatism, out in the sticks. The trouble with the diplomatic model, as described by Bellamy, is that it makes too much virtue out of the petulant failure of the ideological Benthamites, such as Chadwick, to secure all

---

[51]   G. Kearns, P. Laxton and J. Campbell, 'Duncan and the Cholera Test: Public Health in Mid-Nineteenth Century Liverpool', *Transactions of the Historic Society of Lancashire and Cheshire*, 143 (1993), 87–115.

[52]   S. Szreter, *Fertility, Class and Gender in Britain 1860–1914* (Cambridge, 1996), p. 93.

their ends. Rather, we need to reconstruct the distinctive principles and practices which shaped responses both at the centre and in the localities. We need also to acknowledge, in this field, the distinctive political cultures of Whitehall and of individual Town Halls. Historians such as Asa Briggs, E.P. Hennock and Derek Fraser made distinctive local political cultures a central theme in their work, but the extent to which proud city governments formed an effective political network has received less attention. Sanitary reformers in the provinces certainly learned from and relied upon each other.

The Benthamites did, indeed, transform the framework within which central and local government interacted. They brought in techniques of inquiry, inspection and reporting which made the local a feature of national attention in a way it had not been before. But local officers such as Duncan had their own agenda, too, and shuttling between the one and the other, they tried to maintain credit and influence with both under somewhat contradictory pressures. Those pressures allowed Whitehall and Town Hall to learn from and yet frustrate each other.

Acknowledgements

This paper derives from joint work with Paul Laxton and I am very grateful for his help and advice. Hannah Moore, Chris Hamlin, Graham Mooney, Sally Sheard, Chris Philo, Simon Szreter and Naomi Williams have given this research the generous gust of their own ideas and reactions. The Wellcome Trust for the History of Medicine provided funds for our Research Assistant, Joy Campbell, and for Helen Grant to type up Doctor Duncan's letters.

7

Working-class experiences, cholera and public health reform in nineteenth-century Switzerland

Flurin Condrau and Jakob Tanner

Public health reform in Switzerland mostly took place during the second half of the nineteenth century and was generally focused on urban centres. Johanna Bleker and others showed that cities were perceived as an imminent problem of health and order from the late eighteenth century in the discourse of doctors.[1] Together with an increasingly scientific approach to the human body, biological metaphors were applied to urban society: cities were now seen as dirty and, therefore, sick organisms. The accelerated process of urbanisation led, during the second half of the nineteenth century, to an important break in the 'unity' of the city, which began to be divided into areas with different socio-economic and health profiles. Working-class suburbs and the old city centres were increasingly considered as dangerous and as an integral part of a 'monstrous metropolis'.[2] Interestingly, this view of the city was countered by a much more positive interpretation of the urban space. The city was a fascinating and attractive place which offered hitherto unknown and even undreamed-of possibilities and opportunities and a chance for new ways of life. Thus, far from merely being a space within which problems became more ubiquitous, the city promised an alternative and a better way of life for the inhabitants.

In Switzerland, the process of urbanisation, as opposed to the rather idyllic cottage industries, turned into a driving force facilitating the genesis of modern

---

[1]   J. Bleker, 'Die Stadt als Krankheitsfaktor. Eine Analyse ärztlicher Auffassungen im 19. Jahrhundert', *Medizinhistorisches Journal*, 18 (1983), 118–36; F. Walter, *La Suisse urbaine 1750–1959* (Carouge, 1994), pp. 220ff, 319.

[2]   B. Lodewijk, 'Die Stadt als Leviathan. Henry Mayhew und die Londoner Welt', *Historische Anthropologie*, 3 (1995), 460–477; J.V. Pickstone, 'Dearth, Dirt and Fever Epidemics: Rewriting the History of British "Public Health", 1780–1850', in T. Ranger and P. Slack (eds), *Epidemics and Ideas. Essays on the Historical Perception of Pestilence* (Cambridge, 1992), pp. 125–48.

production, the rise of capitalism and today's industrial society.[3] The main characteristic of the expansion of the major Swiss cities during the second half of the nineteenth century was a sudden and rather strict socio-topographical segregation. From the 1890s onwards, the antagonistic city structure was developed by the forced immigration of foreign labour.[4] The market mechanism for condominiums and flats additionally speeded up this process, inasmuch as the low-paid wage-earners who were already confronted with notoriously bad conditions of life had to live in relatively expensive neighbourhoods which in turn made them even poorer, whereas the rich, due to the new mobility, were able to move to affordable areas to occupy a larger chunk of the land.[5]

For obvious reasons urbanisation and overall growth of the major cities contributed to a redefinition of social problems, which in turn raised public health issues. The neighbourhoods of the lower social classes, frequently identical with the old historic centres, suffered from increasingly scarce and crowded residential space and an accumulation of problems relative to food and hygienic conditions.[6] A deterioration of available food due to the increasing commercialisation, and the break-down of the fresh-water supply and the sewage system due to the overuse of ancient infrastructures, increased the 'social inequality of illness and death'.[7] The high mortality found in the 'problematic neighbourhoods' of these burgeoning towns due to the ever-present epidemics of the nineteenth century (smallpox, cholera, typhoid and

---

[3]   Only during the economic upturn, which in the late nineteenth century was supported by new leading sectors of the industrialisation process, did a close coupling between industrialisation and the dynamics of urbanisation happen. Walter, *La Suisse urbaine*, p. 104. Urban spaces quickly became overcrowded. A national census from 1888 shows that in the fifteen largest Swiss cities trade and industry dominated. For a general overview see C. Zimmermann, *Die Zeit der Metropolen. Urbanisierung und Großstadtentwicklung* (Frankfurt, 1996).

[4]   In other European countries the tendency to intra-urban segregation was already apparent at the beginning of the nineteenth century, whereas Switzerland showed a substantial delay in this respect, see Walter, *La Suisse urbaine*, pp. 212, 218.

[5]   B. Fritzsche, 'Mechanismen der sozialen Segregation', in H.-J. Teuteberg (ed.) *Homo habitans. Zur Sozialgeschichte des ländlichen und städtischen Wohnens in der Neuzeit* (Munster, 1985), pp. 155–68.

[6]   In this respect, the following studies are very informative: W. Schüpbach, *Die Bevölkerung der Stadt Luzern 1850–1914. Demographie, Wohnverhältnisse, Hygiene und medizinische Versorgung* (Luzern, 1983); H.P. Bärtschi, *Industrialisierung, Eisenbahnschlachten und Städtebau. Die Entwicklung des Zürcher Industrie- und Arbeiterstadtteils Aussersihl* (Basel, 1983); B. Koller, *'Gesundes Wohnen'. Ein Konstrukt zur Vermittlung bürgerlicher Werte und Verhaltensnormen und seine praktische Umsetzung in der Deutschschweiz 1880–1940* (Zurich, 1995); J. Burnett, *A Social History of Housing 1815–1985* (London, 1985).

[7]   R. Spree, *Health and Social Class in Imperial Germany. A Social History of Mortality, Morbidity and Inequality* (Oxford, 1988).

influenza) and equally omnipresent tuberculosis, were the most brutal manifestation of this situation.[8]

The traditional approach to social history fell short in explaining these diverging aspects in the discourse of experience (economic and cultural chances vs. moral and health dangers of the city) and in the urban environment (class segregation of neighbourhoods) because it was based on the assumption that a city was sufficiently defined as a specific type of urban space, which in turn was a logical consequence of its demographic, epidemiological, economic and social structures. Recent research and the general upswing in studies focusing on the term 'city' in a more linguistic sense suggests, however, that a city is a social environment created by society, which in turn affects society's dynamics of change.[9] Thus, town equals urbanity which in turn consists of a fabric of social customs or practice. The meaning of the perceived entity of 'town' is therefore linked to the social use which may well differ among individuals, groups and classes. Furthermore, there is a paradox arising from the fact that one could produce an image of the town from the perspective of an inhabitant or, as is often the case, as an imaginary phenomenon.[10] Thus, to explain the reproduction of towns and cities the attention has shifted away from economic and material investments more towards collective representations; that is, ideas about the town or the city do not 'reflect' a given social reality but are acquired and changed by society, which includes the people living there. The appropriation of a contextualised way of life is based on these imaginary ideas composed of desires, hopes and fears, which offer certain means of orientation in times of rapid changes in the traditionally family-oriented ways of life.[11] These collective representations affect subjective group, gender and generation-related interpretations of situations alike and require a specific language. The following analysis will focus on the heterogeneous formulation and the varying use of this 'language of disease' in Switzerland during the late nineteenth century. Recent research shows the value of the Swiss case-study as it includes democratic politics, a comparably early and strong process of industrialisation and an overall picture which is easier to grasp than, say, in Germany.[12] The first section will deal mainly with the general links between

---

[8]   F. Condrau, 'Soziale Ungleichheit vor Cholera und ihre Wahrnehmung durch Zürichs Ärzteschaft (1850–1870)', *Medizin, Gesellschaft und Geschichte. Jahrbuch der Robert Bosch Stiftung für die Geschichte der Medizin*, 12 (1994), 75–100.

[9]   Walter, *La Suisse urbaine*.

[10]   This leads us back to the aforementioned issue of cities and towns in the medical discourse.

[11]   R. Chartier, 'Die Welt als Repräsentation', in M. Middell and S. Sammler (eds), *Alles Gewordene hat Geschichte. Die Schule der Annales in ihren Texten 1929–1992* (Leipzig, 1994), pp. 320–47.

[12]   F. Condrau, 'Cholera und Sozialer Wandel. Die Schweiz als Beispiel', in J. Vögele (ed.), *Stadt, Krankheit und Tod. Stadtischen Gesundheitsvarhattuisse während der Epidemiologischen Transition* (Berlin, 2000) pp. 189–208.

urban conditions, public health and scientific debates; the second section shifts attention towards the language of medical doctors during two cholera epidemics in Zurich; the third section will concentrate on the political conflicts in relation to the cholera epidemic of 1867, whereas the fourth and last section will focus on working-class experience and popular tales which were again linked to class, gender, age and regional customs.

Scientific debates and the urban space

The nineteenth century is usually characterised by an increasingly medico-scientific approach to society and social problems which, in turn, created a new fabric of knowledge and thus allowed changes in the power structure and strategies of intervention. Homogenising disciplinary tendencies 'from above' and rather disparate expectations and attitudes 'from below' affected each other and resulted in a 'modernisation' of health-related attitudes and the handling of diseases.[13] In the burgeoning industrial centres, health was now perceived as a public problem to be tackled. In these new urban ways of life, the assurance of 'public health' had to be adjusted to the increasing mobility of people, and the general growth of urban areas required integration into the well-known routines of collective-space administration. Thus, the urban environment became a laboratory to test new forms of public health approaches within the local government.[14]

The focus on the language of disease can explain the imaginary 'mapping' of urban space as an expression of semantic dichotomisations. In particular in the nineteenth century, the discussion of health and disease was strongly structured by such binary and relational antonyms. The most prominent of these was the differentiation between town and countryside. It was further enriched by opposites such as healthy versus ill, musty versus fresh, dark versus light, spoiled versus pure, artificial versus natural, dirty versus clean, confused versus clear, hectic versus calm, untidy versus tidy, and so on. To understand public health movements during the nineteenth century Mary Douglas suggested these paired terms had converged to create an image of order which then became a positive acquisition and subsequently legitimised action aimed at preserving or restoring the new order: 'Dirt is essentially disorder ... Dirt offends against order. Eliminating it is not a negative movement, but a positive effort to

---

[13]   A. Labisch, *Homo Hygienicus. Gesundheit und Medizin in der Neuzeit* (Frankfurt, 1992).

[14]   B. Witzler, *Großstadt und Hygiene. Kommunale Gesundheitspolitik in der Epoche der Urbanisierung* (Stuttgart, 1995); P. Münch, *Stadthygiene im 19. und 20. Jahrhundert. Die Wasserversorgung, Abwasser- und Abfallbeseitigung unter besonderer Berücksichtigung Münchens* (Göttingen, 1993).

organise the environment'.[15] This 'elimination' was at first a demand made plausible by the new debate on the endangering of order and health by lack of morals and dirt. The town was now perceived as an entity which tended to be both endangered and dangerous. This was exemplified by the publication in 1872 of political economist Victor Böhmert's study on the 'Swiss Workers' Situation in the Last Ten Years' which had been commissioned by the Schweizerische Gemeinnützige Gesellschaft (a Swiss charity). This study linked the terminology of socio-cultural changes in industrial society, upheavals within the working classes and health-endangering factors.[16] Along with political crisis, wars, transport and communication innovations, and a concomitant liberation of politics and economy, Böhmert averred that 'the revival of socialist theories and plots ... generated an enormous upheaval of the working classes and a profound leavening process'. Nevertheless, he suggested that Switzerland with its still largely rural population, limited landed property and the thriftiness of its population had shown itself remarkably resistant against the political agitation of the left. Böhmert used medical terms to plead for a general, preventive hygienics to replace a purely curative approach: 'Just as in medicine and public health care, the so-called preventive, prophylactic measures and provisions preventing social crises are much more important for the social health care of the population than the more often than not questionable medicines employed to heal already existing diseases'.[17] This statement shows the increasing self-confidence of a closely-knit community of scientific experts who based their findings on the assumption that social problems could be solved by rational measures and efficient policy-making within the existing social system.

Urbanisation was often accompanied by the formation of an organised labour movement.[18] In Switzerland, citizens began to conjure up the 'danger from below' and to plan practical measures to assure law and order. Given the constant class struggle, the rather alarmist rhetoric intensified. In the second half of the 1880s, the increasingly militant attitude of the workers led to a dramatic deterioration of relations between the urban élite and the working classes and an equally increasing escalation of conflicts within the urban space.[19] Repression and reform were the two complementary strategies used to

---

[15]   M. Douglas, *Purity and Danger. An Analysis of the Concepts of Pollution and Taboo* (London, 1994), p. 2.
[16]   V. Böhmert, *Schweizerische Arbeiter-Verhältnisse in den letzten zehn Jahren* (Zurich, 1872).
[17]   Ibid., p.33.
[18]   R.J. Evans, *Death in Hamburg. Society and Politics in the Cholera Years 1830–1910* (Oxford, 1987).
[19]   Walter, *La Suisse urbaine*, p. 242. See also H. Hirter, 'Streiks 1880–1914', in E. Gruner (ed.), *Arbeiterschaft und Wirtschaft in der Schweiz 1880–1914*, vol. 2/2, Gewerkschaften und Arbeitgeber auf dem Arbeitsmarkt (Zurich, 1988).

answer to these challenges. In most towns, the police force was increased, and the middle classes became more aware of the poor conditions of life and the supply problems which the lower classes were subjected to. Here, the dichotomous categories of 'clean' and 'dirty' developed their full potential as distinctions of class: the forced perception of dirt as disorder by the middle classes and scientific experts was primarily an expression of this new awareness of a sense of order based on cleanliness. In Switzerland, the discussion of social reforms was also characterised by a symbolic identification with the extreme of that being criticised. Qualifications such as 'dirty', 'reeking' and 'unhygienic' were semantic contrasts set against the middle-class way of life.[20] Gerd Göckenjan exaggerated this hypothesis stating that the history of health definitions was at the same time 'a history of the social obsessions of the middle classes ... The topic of health condenses the fears and hopes of a permanently insecure world'.[21] The fact that a scientific analysis of problems, bourgeois snobbery, and fear of the 'mob' and epidemics had turned into a close symbiosis was the most important issue. However, these new patterns of interpretation were not continuously adopted, but rather accepted in times of crises and at turning points which allowed these new approaches and solutions to be implemented.

Cholera and poverty in the medical discourse in Zurich

We will now turn to the cholera epidemic which broke out in Zurich in the summer of 1867 and characterised just such a turning point. Its perception was still strongly influenced by the experience of urban authorities and the population during the first cholera epidemic of 1855. The demographic significance of the epidemic in the sense of a mortality crisis was not of paramount importance: all in all, there were 481 victims, which equalled 78 dead per 100,000 population. Contemporaries however, noted that mortality was highest in the rapidly spreading working-class suburbs that had come into existence at the perimeter of Zurich. Aussersihl was the worst hit in absolute number of cases. This rather preoccupied people, and is a good example of the idea that absolute numbers were often more important to the directly affected than any (relative) mortality rates.[22] In 1855, it had still been possible to efficiently and calmly control the cholera epidemic with the help of traditional quarantines. Twelve years later, the authorities soon declared themselves overwhelmed. Traditional measures now contrasted all too visibly with the

---

[20]   Evans, *Death in Hamburg*, p. 178.
[21]   G. Göckenjan, *Kurieren und Staat machen. Gesundheit und Medizin in der bürgerlichen Welt* (Frankfurt, 1985), p. 15.
[22]   Condrau, 'Soziale Ungleichheit', 77–85.

liberal imperatives of industrial transport and economy which were based on a free circulation of people and goods.

Countless people ignored police orders meant to fight the epidemic and left their houses, which led to punitive measures. In court, they stated that they had not only suffered terrible losses from the cholera but also enormous material disadvantages because of the quarantine measures: 'indem uns durch diese wenn auch nothwendigen Massregeln, unser Verdienst gänzlich abgebrochen wird und wir kein Vermögen besitzen um unsere Familien ohne diesen täglichen Verdienst zu unterhalten'.[23] For them, it didn't really matter whether they were struck by cholera or starved by the police forces. Others initiated large damage claims against the medical authorities which caused severe financial problems for the latter. Typically, it was an industrialist and employer, the owner of the Escher-Wyss AG engineering works, who opposed the orders of district physician Dr Zehnder and threatened to shut down his factory if the authorities actually interfered in his affairs using the justification of epidemiological measures. It is interesting to see that all Zehnder asked Escher and Wyss to do was a refurbishment of the toilets and bathrooms. Escher and Wyss's retort was that a few cases of cholera would be easier to bear than the cost of the proposed hygienic measures: 'Da eine solche Massregel der gänzlichen Arbeitseinstellung in unseren Werkstätten gleichkkäme ... müssten wir solches für eine Ausschreitung des Amtseifers halten'.[24] People were so unconvinced that all measures to fight the epidemic were abandoned shortly after it had broken out in spite of the district physician's explicit protest. This came at a time, moreover, when it was not yet clear whether the epidemic would actually prove more serious than the one of 1855.[25] Without being able to offer a reasonable alternative strategy to fight the cholera epidemic, the administration had to give up the 'old' measures. Interestingly, the medically-informed quarantine measures were dropped because they threatened to have worse consequences for a liberal society than the epidemic itself.

The 1867 epidemic not only hampered any attempts at quarantine, but changed the way the disease and above all those infected were perceived. A new view of poverty and a new interpretation of the 'social question' gained increasing acceptance.[26] During the 1855 epidemic, district physician Johann Jacob Schrämli was still convinced that the 'cholera miasma' was only able to

---

[23] Witwe Hammer und Mitunterzeichnende an Präsident der Polizeikommission Römer (letter to the president of the police council), 1.9.1867, in Stadtarchiv Zurich (StaZ), VFc03.

[24] Escher-Wyss & Co. an Präsident der Polizeikommission Römer (letter to the president of the police council), 31.8.1867, in Stadtarchiv Zurich (StaZ), VFc01:2.

[25] Protocoll der Medicinaldirection und des Medicinalrathes (minutes of the local sanitary authorities), 30.8.1867, in Staatsarchiv Zurich (StaZ), SS 4:17.

[26] Condrau, 'Soziale Ungleichheit', 88–93; see also J.V. Pickstone, 'Ferriar's Fever to Kay's Cholera: Disease and Social Structure in Cottonopolis', *History of Science*, 22 (1984), 401–19.

generate the disease in the 'poorly' and 'unfit-to-work' poor. Those poor were then presumed to infect the more 'robust' and 'healthy'.[27] The director of the medical department of the Zurich Cantonal Hospital, Professor Dr Hermann Lebert, believed it was the life of excess led by the poor and their lack of confidence in physicians which were responsible for the cholera outbreak.[28] Lebert and Schrämli, both leading physicians at the time of the first cholera epidemic in Zurich, are typical examples of what Richard Evans called 'moralistic miasmaticians'.[29] Indeed, the description of the disease (miasma) and the concomitant recriminations (attribution of fault) developed hand in hand.

During and following the 1867 epidemic, the focus of attention shifted. The moralising allocation of fault to suspicious and deviant individuals was given up in favour of socio-topographic explanations. Discussions focused on urban findings and, in particular, the working-class suburb of Aussersihl as well as some typical workers and dwellings in the old centre of town (Niederdorf). On the one hand, the epidemic was much more severe in certain neighbourhoods; on the other hand, it hit the poor within these neighbourhoods most severely. This part of the population was said to 'have to fight very hard against misery and poverty'. Zehnder critised the overcrowded accommodation. The building standards of houses were below par and the sewerage system downright catastrophic.[30] The medical director of the Zurich Cantonal Hospital, Professor Anton Biermer, acknowledged: 'Our patients are, with a very few exceptions, from the working classes and all kinds of professions ... Of the female patients, most are workers, wives, unmarried factory workers, and maids'.[31] It is obvious that Biermer abandoned the idea of a moral classification for cholera victims and instead identified the labouring poor as the core problem group for urban society. The perception of poverty had changed and led to an awareness of the social opposites within the city as the real problem. It led away from the moralistic theory of miasmas to an empirical understanding of social questions which physicians, however, tended to translate in a somewhat socio-technical manner into a question of hygienic infrastructure and thus into an argument to sanitise the town.

---

[27]   J. J. Schrämli, *Bezirksärztlicher Bericht über die Choleraepidemie des Bezirkes Zürich im Herbst 1855* (Zürich, 1856), pp. 12–15.

[28]   H. Lebert, *Die Cholera in der Schweiz und das über dieselbe im Züricher Kantons-Spital beobachtete. Ein Bericht an die Medizinaldirektion* (Frankfurt, 1856), p. 19.

[29]   Evans, *Death in Hamburg*, p. 248.

[30]   C. Zehnder, *Bericht über die Choleraepidemie des Jahres 1867 im Kanton Zürich* (Zurich, 1871), p. 18f.

[31]   A. Biermer, 'Mittheilungen über die medizinische Klinik', in *Jahresbericht über die Verwaltung des Medizinalwesens, die öffentlichen Krankenanstalten und den allgemeinen Gesundheitszustand des Kantons Zürich im Jahre 1867 nebst Mittheilungen aus der Praxis der Aerzte und Thierärzte erstattet von der Direktion der Medizinalangelegenheiten* (Zurich, 1869), p. 29.

Cholera and the political discourse in Zurich

The changing attitudes of the physicians interpreting the *status quo* in Zurich were closely linked to the changing scientific concept of how to fight diseases. By itself, this is not yet a satisfactory explanation, though, for it is merely shifting the problem from the explanation of the strategies developed to fight cholera to an explanation of changing perceptions of cholera. However, for both aspects, it may have been crucial that the 1867 cholera epidemic in Zurich was the result of a more extensive crisis caused by something altogether different.

In the second half of the 1860s, after long years of political stability, the canton of Zurich suffered a severe political crisis, which was linked to the so-called 'democratic movement'.[32] It was caused by the question of whether the political system could conceivably be reformed and how this might be achieved. This put the representative democracy, the established constitution since 1848, under attack. The reformers demanded the introduction of non-direct democratic elements, reasoning that the people were no longer willing to be governed by 'state, railway, and banking barons'.[33] Within the context of this radical political climate, the outbreak of the cholera epidemic gained new importance. It was burdened by metaphors and understood to be an expression of a 'sick system'. 'Physical putrefaction developed out of political rot, and that's why cholera has come to Zurich', a leftist's pamphlet proclaimed.[34] Disease became a political problem which was taken up by the democratic movement and other agitators and used to attack the liberal government. There is an interesting difference between the formulas 'disease as political problem' and 'disease as problem for politics'. The former refers to the object of the political process, pointing out that disease has been recognised as a political problem, while the latter considers disease as capital in the political process which can be used to achieve other political goals. Karl Bürkli, a leading democrat, established a striking analogy between the political system and the cholera epidemic at the Landsgemeinde in Zurich on 15 December 1867:

> I define *system* as the negative influence of economic interest and economy, above all that of the North-Eastern Railways as headquarters, the Credit Suisse, many important industrialists, government-clerks, and

[32]   M. Schaffner, *Die demokratische Bewegung der 1860er Jahre. Beschreibung und Erklärung der Zürcher Volksbewegung von 1867* (Basel, 1982).

[33]   The leading liberal politician Alfred Escher was a Member of Parliament. He was also at the head of some of the most important enterprises of the time including the *Schweizerische Nordostbahn* (founded in 1853) and the *Credit Suisse* (founded in 1857); see Schaffner, *Bewegung*, p. 27.

[34]   La Suisse Radicale, quoted in G.A. Craig, *Geld und Geist. Zürich im Zeitalter des Liberalismus 1830–1869* (Munich, 1988), p. 268.

the freemasons. The system can, as cholera, not be easily defined though you feel it in your very bones ... we now have to topple a new, rampant but illegal financial aristocracy.[35]

The cholera epidemic not only intensified the general tone of political debates but developed into an indicator of social evils which the liberal government seemed to be unable to find an answer to. In fact, the disease undermined the credibility or rather the trustworthiness of the political system and thus substantially contributed to its downfall.[36]

Between 1863 and 1876, Zurich's economy was hit by a steep downtrend. More than a decade after the railway boom, in the autumn and winter of 1867–68, investments hit an all-time low.[37] Agriculture also suffered a downturn. The scarcity of capital, sinking prices for wheat and the bad harvests of 1866 and 1867 ruined many small and medium-sized businesses and farms or got them into debt with the banks.[38] Finally, the textile industry in the Zurich Oberland suffered an unprecedented decline in orders.[39] This crisis had begun without the influence of cholera. The epidemic, however, helped people perceive and dramatise it. It made its contemporaries aware of the danger and the epidemic aspect of the crisis more visible and felt. It also increased the latent conflict between the rapidly expanding industrial and administrative centre in Zurich and the largely agricultural countryside. Food supply for Zurich became a problem because the inhabitants of several smaller towns and villages were forbidden to travel to Zurich and attempted to hassle arriving travellers (in particular traders from Zurich) by imposing quarantine measures on them.[40] It became an administrative nightmare to supply the town from its environs, and

---

[35]   S. Bleuler-Hausheer, *Aktenstücke aus der Zürcherischen Revisionsbewegung. Vollständige Sammlung der Landsgemeinde-Reden, Proklamation des Kantonalkomités und der Abstimmungsresultate* (Winterthur, 1868), p. 11; see also D. Decurtins and S. Grossmann, 'Die Bedeutung kommunikativer Vernetzung für die Gründung der Zürcher Kantonalbank 1870', in Y. Cassis and J. Tanner (eds), *Bankensystem und Geldpolitik in der Schweiz* (Zurich, 1993), p. 108.

[36]   See K. Dändliker, *Geschichte der Stadt und des Kantons Zürich*. vol. 3: Von 1712 bis zur Gegenwart (Zurich, 1912), pp. 378f.

[37]   H. Siegenthaler, 'Die Schweiz 1850–1914', in W. Fischer (ed.), *Europäische Wirtschafts- und Sozialgeschichte von der Mitte des 19. Jahrhunderts bis zum Ersten Weltkrieg, Europäische Wirtschafts- und Sozialgeschichte vol. 5* (Stuttgart, 1987), pp. 443–73.

[38]   P. Gilg, *Die Entstehung der demokratischen Bewegung und die soziale Frage. Die sozialen Ideen und Postulate der deutschschweizerischen Demokraten in den frühen 60er Jahren des 19. Jahrhunderts* (Zurich, DPhil thesis, 1951), p. 71; Schaffner, *Bewegung*, pp. 102–6.

[39]   Schaffner, *Bewegung*, p. 111.

[40]   Schreiben der Direction der Justiz des eidgenössischen Standes Zürich an die Statthalterämter (letter of Department of Justice of the Canton Zurich to the governor's office), in Staatsarchiv Zurich (StaZ), SS 119:1.

soup kitchens had to be opened in town to feed the population. A witness to these times recalls:

> Those who visited Zurich in the autumn of 1867 felt they entered an enormous morgue. The once lively town was silent, no songs and no pleasures were to be had, streets were laid waste and silent, pubs were empty, and where there used to be wonderful music, where the business of the exchange once had enlivened the halls of the Tonhalle, only the long rows of beds of hospitals marked by misery could be seen.[41]

Beyond the drama the author evokes with these lines, he also documents that the already weakened economy of the town was virtually paralysed by the cholera epidemic. It was not so much the cholera itself but the reaction of people to it which affected the economy. Thus, the epidemic increased people's awareness of the economic crisis.

Popular tales and working-class cholera experience

Modern medical knowledge of the importance of a hygienic infrastructure, and the new concepts of diseases and illness discussed by licensed physicians, also affected the popular image of the danger the epidemic represented. At the same time, social customs which made no sense from the point of view of enlightened science and were thus fought as the superstitious relics of earlier times, were still practised by large parts of the population. The following example shows how the Zurich cholera epidemic of 1867 was perceived by a child. The author, Verena Conzett, a renowned social reformer and wife of a well-known social democrat, published her autobiography in 1929 and told how she got to know about cholera as a small child in the 'desolate' and 'practically deserted' town of Zurich. Everywhere, children stood side by side, looking down, without playing as they were wont to do.

> I was curious, climbed a hillock, and saw how all the boys and girls pulled small white pouches from underneath their clothes, some hastily, others more circumspectly. They compared them as to the shape and the fineness of the linen. Helen Müller proudly stated: 'Look, my pouch has a silk ribbon', and Hansruedeli, the smallest of all my schoolmates, called out: 'And mine has a beautiful blue string!'

Questioned by Verena Conzett, who was the same age, as to why the small pouches were of such paramount importance to them, her schoolmates reacted rather grumpily: 'Those are amulets and we wear them because of the cholera!

---

[41]   T. Koller quoted by Craig, *Geld*, p. 267f.

... Why – does Vreneli [Verena] truly ignore that we have cholera in Zurich?'
Verena Conzett came to understand that 'cholera was a terribly evil woman – a
terrifying black woman who killed people, strangling them, and that only those
wearing such an amulet were safe from her'. The narrator then recalled upon
her return to the classroom that she had already once before seen this 'terrible
Madam Cholera':

> Close to our flat was the old lunatic asylum ... One day, when I was in
> the courtyard, a woman with straggling hair came running; she shouted
> and tried to pounce on those present. Wardens hurried over and tried to
> subdue her, but she went berserk and hit everything in sight, and it
> required a protracted struggle to take her back. I was all pale and
> trembling when I returned ...[42]

When school was out, Verena Conzett ran home and told her mother about this
truly terrible thing: 'Why, Vreneli, what stories you tell; that's not true, you
know. There is no Madam Cholera! Just think, if such a terrible woman really
existed, the police would long ago have jailed her'. The mother thereupon
explained that cholera was a disease and that only prayers helped keep it at bay.
As an adult, the author then recalled her childhood environment: the narrow,
high houses, the dark flats never touched by a even a single ray of sun, and the
'smelly, musty air' of the rooms. 'Most people who lived in the narrow alleys
of Zurich at the time suffered similar or worse conditions. No wonder then that
cholera was able to hold its sway everywhere given such unsanitary
conditions.'[43] This epidemiological statement of the now adult author, who
assumes the scientific and enlightened part of this communication, was,
however, superimposed on memories of her childhood. Verena Conzett
described how, upon her mother's advice, she began to pray feverishly, though
she was unable 'to master her fear of "Madam Cholera" in spite of all my
parents and my older sisters said ....Whenever I climbed up or down our dark
flights of stairs, I felt her close, felt her breath touch me and her bony hand
grasp me. I used to run down these stairs driven by pure fright'. The woman
waiting behind every corner remained a constant presence in the world of the
child – only the retrospective tale of the now grown-up Verena Conzett turned
it into an enlightened tale of the tribulations caused by these childhood
imaginings.

---

[42]   V. Conzett, *Erstrebtes und Erlebtes. Ein Stück Zeitgeschichte* (Leipzig, 1929), pp.
13ff.
[43]   Ibid., p. 19.

Conclusion

The rationalisation process shown by this story may be interpreted as part of a predominant tendency to turn health and illness into scientific facts and define the concomitant problems. Due to a general urban-health policy based on and legitimised by scientific interpretations, the last third of the nineteenth century was characterised by expensive investments in infrastructures such as urban water supply and sewerage systems.

Although the bio-cyclical behaviour of pathogens had already been experimentally described in the two preceding decades, and the existence of micro-organisms as necessary if not sufficient cause of diseases was known, the miasma theory still governed even 'updated' official measures until the 1880s. Far from being a precise or even limited way to describe diseases and epidemics, it nevertheless provided the preconditions to convey political news. On the one hand, it allowed a link to be established between 'sources of danger', the lower social classes, the danger of epidemics, and revolutionary infection. It also imposed the necessity to control this threat to urban and wider society by reforms and, in particular, socio-hygienic information and infrastructural measures. On the other hand, it linked sick bodies to a sick system and helped to model the semantics of an attempt at urban political reform. In both cases, the language of illness supported the efforts of hygienic experts who were convinced an increased political intervention in urban society would improve social conditions.

The long and frequently quite scurrilous discussion led by the exponents of the miasma theory and those postulating a system of contagion was ultimately won by the latter. The change of paradigm linked to the names of Robert Koch and Louis Pasteur was not a clear break and caused some rather ambivalent reactions. It promoted a development which might be defined as a politicisation of health, disease and health care. And, while the labour movement considered the most effective remedial approach to social problems and any factors rendering people ill to be an increase in wages and a reduction in working times, the middle classes (for once supported by the left) proposed a 'right to be ill' guaranteed by public health insurance.[44] At the same time, the fight against the 'invisible monster'[45] now entered a new stage, not least in its linguistic expression.[46] The ill were no longer the centre of medical attention. Bacteria and viruses took their place, were personalised synonymously with the

---

[44]   C. Herzlich and J. Pierret, *Kranke gestern, Kranke heute: die Gesellschaft und das Leiden* (Munich, 1991), pp. 67ff.

[45]   G. Vigarello, *Le propre et le sale. L'hygiene du corps depuis le Moyen Age* (Paris, 1985) pp. 218ff; see also G. Vigarello, *Le sain et le malsain. Santé et mieux-être depuis le Moyen Age* (Paris, 1993).

[46]   C. Gradmann, 'Bakterien, Krankheit und Krieg. Bakteriologie und politische Sprache im Deutschen Kaiserreich', *Berichte zur Wissenschaftsgeschichte*, 19 (1996), 81–94.

respective diseases and declared the enemies of humanity. This furthered the use of aggressive war metaphors: the 'annihilation of pathogens' was increasingly linked to the 'health of the public body' and the 'purity of race' and thus made subservient to the legitimisation of these political concepts of the enemy. This popular scientific battle language culminated in the anti-Semitic and anti-gypsy movement. It contributed to the consolidation of those prejudices which were to play such a devastating role in the history of the twentieth century. If we were not sensible to the dangers of biologising an idea, we might say that the 'language of disease' had quite precariously fallen 'ill' in the late nineteenth century, too.

8

Public health discourses in Birmingham and Gothenburg, 1890–1920

Marjaana Niemi

By the early twentieth century, urban health authorities were accustomed to political criticism. The question which frequently sparked fierce political controversy in both British and Swedish cities was defective housing. In the eyes of some property owners, public health measures that aimed to alleviate housing problems were only 'thinly disguised weapons of a great Socialistic raid upon property'. Left-wing critics, for their part, accused health officials of being cowards who did not dare to touch 'the pockets of the owners of ... vile slums'.[1] Similarly, health issues concerning reproduction and sex often inspired heated debates and angry protests. The opponents of birth control insisted that public health experts and executives should adhere to their view and save society from moral collapse, whereas the advocates urged them to provide birth control advice and save thousands of women from serious health problems.[2] In these cases, health authorities could not win. If they did nothing, they laid themselves open to charges of inaction and political bias; if they did something they were frequently criticised for going too far and, again, serving political ends. Their stance was always contested, no matter how much scientific evidence they produced to support it.

---

[1]   See, for example, Birmingham Public Record Office (hereafter BPRO), Birmingham Public Health Committee (PHC), minutes 28. 2. 1913 item 1224; A. Gough, *Objections to the Housing and Town-Planning Bill of the Right Honourable John Burns and to the Housing of the Working Classes Bill Introduced by Mr. Bowerman, With Birmingham's Experience of the Housing Acts* (Birmingham, 1908), p. 2; *Göteborgs Stadsfullmäktiges Handlingar* (hereafter *GSH*) 1913:337; 1923:328 and minutes 13. 9. 1923 and discussion; G. Göthlin, 'Några bostadshygieniska reformkrav', Göteborgs Läkaresällskaps förhandlingar 13. 9., *Hygiea* lxxix (1917), 1151–69.

[2]   'Kvinnokongressen i Stockholm', *Ny Tid* 7. 8. 1908; 'Sexuell hygien. Dr. Alma Sundqvists föredrag å soc.dem. kvinnokongressen', *Ny Tid* 11. 8. 1908; 'Det tomma intet', *Ny Tid* 9. 5. 1910; 'Mot ofruktsamhetspropagandan. Gårdagens stora opinionsmöte', *Göteborgs-Posten* 9. 5. 1910; (BPRO) Birmingham Maternity and Child Welfare Committee, minutes 5. 3. 1931 item 585; 13. 3. 1931 item 590.

Yet the majority of public health questions aroused neither political anger nor moral uproar. Health authorities in Britain and Sweden were clearly successful in conveying the impression that, in most cases, their analysis of urban health problems was scientific and thus value-free and objective. The statistical tables, charts and maps which health officials used to illustrate public health questions were usually accepted as unproblematic and neutral. Reports in which they defined health problems by utilising the latest findings of contemporary science were not seriously questioned. However, public health campaigns had many national and local characteristics which clearly show that health authorities had a considerable degree of latitude when it came to defining urban health problems. Their statistical tables concealed as much as they revealed, and their reports emphasised some research findings and were silent on others. By comparing the ways in which the authorities analysed and defined problems of public health in the second cities of Britain and Sweden (Birmingham and Gothenburg) this study examines the political and social aims advanced by the allegedly neutral language of urban public health reform.

Recent debates about the socio-cultural dimensions of medicine and health care have provided useful insights into the theme of alleged neutrality. Particularly important is the recognition that basic social relations such as capitalist economic arrangements, the family system and the nation state have always shaped our knowledge about health and illness. Hence, the identification of a collective well-being with the market economy and family system has been implicit in basically all definitions of public health problems and in responses to them.[3] Building on these insights, this chapter looks at the role which 'scientific' public health policy played in urban politics and governance in the early twentieth century. It is argued here that the ways in which health authorities defined environmental problems or 'social diseases' such as tuberculosis, infant mortality and venereal diseases did not only help to maintain the capitalist economic system and the family in general, but they also served to legitimate different national and local arrangements in the fields of economy, politics and morals. In illustrating and analysing urban health problems – in making the unknown known – authorities reinforced, both

---

[3]   A. Sears, '"To teach them how to live". The politics of public health from tuberculosis to AIDS', *Journal of Historical Sociology*, 5 (1992), 61–83; R. N. Proctor, *Cancer Wars. How Politics Shape What We Know and Don't Know About Cancer* (New York, 1995); L. Jordanova, 'The social construction of medical knowledge', *Social History of Medicine*, 8 (1995), 361–81; G. Kearns, 'Tuberculosis and the medicalisation of British society, 1880–1920', in J. Woodward and R. Jütte (eds), *Coping with Sickness. Historical Aspects of Health Care in a European Perspective* (Sheffield, 1995), pp. 147–70; H. Waitzkin, 'A critical theory of medical discourse: ideology, social control, and the processing of social context in medical encounters', *Journal of Health and Social Behaviour*, 30 (1989), 220–39; B. Harrison, 'Women and health', in J. Purvis (ed.), *Women's History: Britain, 1850–1945 An Introduction* (London, 1995), pp. 157–92.

wittingly and unwittingly, existing relationships of power and structures of inequality.[4]

This chapter begins by discussing the ways in which health authorities 'mapped' cities in the late nineteenth and early twentieth centuries, and the political assumptions underlying these maps. In Birmingham, where suburbs – or more precisely the interdependent relationship of slums and suburbs – crucially contributed to the political and economic power of the middle class, the definition of public health problems, both in the nineteenth century and early twentieth century, served to reinforce the impression of a segregated city. In Gothenburg, where the middle class built its economic and political power largely on factors other than social segregation, the definitions of urban health problems throughout the period reviewed here were constructed to answer the 'needs' of a socially mixed town.[5] The chapter then looks at the basic tenets of the anti-tuberculosis campaigns in Birmingham and Gothenburg and in particular the ways in which the rights and responsibilities of the healthy, the sick and the medical profession were defined in these campaigns. In both Birmingham and Gothenburg, health authorities made a concerted effort to show that the policy they pursued was firmly anchored to 'accurate' scientific knowledge. What this study illustrates, however, is that the health authorities tended to take for granted aspects of the new theories that supported their preconceptions about the problem, and they selectively ignored research findings that challenged their assumptions. In Birmingham, the anti-tuberculosis campaign was marked by health authorities' determination to seek both prevention and cure by transforming people's attitudes and behaviour. In Gothenburg, by contrast, the municipal tuberculosis scheme was shaped by the belief that the medical profession would provide a cure or at least prevent the spread of the disease.

The extent to which political aims, moral judgements and professional aspirations were justified by appeals to the authority of 'value-free' science is

---

[4]   For further discussion, see M. Niemi, 'Health, Experts and the Politics of Knowledge. Britain and Sweden 1900–1940' (unpublished PhD thesis, University of Leicester, 1999). See also, for example, J.V. Pickstone, 'Introduction', and M. Worboys, 'The sanatorium treatment for consumption in Britain, 1890–1914', in J. V. Pickstone (ed.), *Medical Innovations in Historical Perspective* (London, 1992), pp. 1–16, 47–71.

[5]   For further discussion about the interdependent relationship of slums and suburbs in Britain, see H.J. Dyos and D.A. Reeder, 'Slums and suburbs', in H.J. Dyos and M. Wolff (eds), *The Victorian City. Images and Realities* Vol. I (London, 1973), pp. 359–86. For residential segregation in Gothenburg, see H. Wallqvist, *Bostadsförhållandena för de mindre bemedlade i Göteborg* (Stockholm, 1891), pp. 4–11, 72–5; M. Åberg, *En fråga om klass? Borgarklass och industriellt företagande i Göteborg, 1850–1914* (Gothenburg, 1991), pp. 132–7; G. Lönnroth, 'Stadsbilden – praktfulla palats och usla kåkar', *För hundra år sedan – skildringar från Göteborgs 1880-tal* (Gothengurg, 1984), pp. 27–62. For the 'mapping' of cities, see C. Topalov, 'The city as terra incognita: Charles Booth's poverty survey and the people of London, 1886–1891', *Planning Perspectives*, 8 (1993), 394–425.

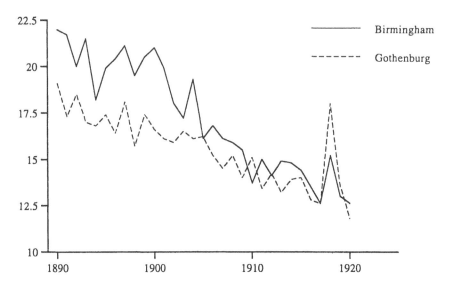

Figure 8.1: Crude death rates in Birmingham and Gothenburg, 1890–1920

Sources: *Annual Report of the Medical Officer of Health for Birmingham for 1910*, 11; *for 1938*, 254; *Statistisk årsbok för Göteborg 1939*, 21–2.

sharply revealed by examining policies pursued by health officials who had access to the same body of medical and scientific knowledge. The British and Swedish public health officials were part of one public health community, enjoying close links, attending the same international conferences and contributing to the same journals.[6] In both Birmingham and Gothenburg, health authorities claimed firm scientific grounds as the basis for their programmes.

---

[6]   In both Birmingham and Gothenburg, public health officials had an active interest in, for example, the international infant welfare and anti-tuberculosis movements. In Gothenburg in particular, study tours to Germany, Britain and France, synopses of 'essential' scientific literature and surveys cataloguing measures taken in other countries were an integral component of the decision-making process. In Birmingham, international contacts played a less important role in the day-to-day policy-making. However, in constructing housing policies, anti-tuberculosis schemes and infant welfare programmes, public health officials contributed to the international debate about these questions and imported ideas from the international arena and in particular from Germany, France, Denmark, Sweden and the United States. Moreover, both Dr John Robertson (the Medical Officer of Health for Birmingham for 1904–27) and Dr Karl Gezelius (the First City Phycisian for Gothenburg for 1901–31) made long study trips to the Continent in the late nineteenth century. See, Niemi, 'Health, Experts and the Politics of Knowledge', ch. 3.

In fact they saw themselves as the leading edge of a new era of health policy which would promote well-being by providing scientific solutions to social and health problems. Furthermore, the problems they dealt with were often very similar. Birmingham and Gothenburg were both industrial cities, with growing populations and expanding economies. The crude death rates for these cities were at the same level, especially in the early twentieth century (Figure 8.1), and in a wider European context both Birmingham and Gothenburg were relatively healthy industrial centres. On the basis of these factors, one could assume that the public health policies pursued by the Birmingham and Gothenburg authorities would have been relatively close to each other. Yet they were often strikingly different and these differences were not necessarily related to the severity of a specific problem such as infant mortality or tuberculosis. The aim of this chapter is to examine some of these differences and to discuss how the approaches chosen by the Birmingham and Gothenburg authorities were shaped by the social, moral and political cultures within which they worked.

This study does not argue that health authorities abused science to advance political aims. Nor does it suggest that they could have used science in a better, apolitical way. The approach of this type would imply that there were value-free scientific theories or approaches which some right-minded, enlightened health authorities could have used to the 'real' benefit of the whole community. This certainly was not the case: all scientific knowledge was affected by political and social concerns, but by looking at the ways in which the Birmingham and Gothenburg health authorities analysed health problems, this study examines a process whereby power structures were legitimated in urban societies.[7]

Mapping the city

In Birmingham, health and sanitary problems received little systematic attention from local authorities before the appointment of the Medical Officer of Health (MOH) in 1873. Birmingham made this move a quarter of a century later than the pioneers, Liverpool, Leicester and London, and even in the early 1870s a large number of Birmingham policy-makers were of the opinion that a medical officer was a luxury they could not afford. Central government showed how little sympathy it had with this kind of view by making the appointment of

---

[7]   For criticism of the use/abuse model, see L. Jordanova, *Sexual Visions. Images of Gender in Science and Medicine Between the Eighteenth and Twentieth Centuries* (New York, 1989), pp. 15–16; *idem*, 'The social construction', p. 367; M. Tiles, 'A science of Mars or of Venus', *Philosophy*, 62 (1987), 293–306.

an MOH obligatory in 1872.[8] Dr Alfred Hill, who was appointed as the Birmingham MOH, devoted the first ten years of his tenure to bringing the local public health administration and sanitary policy into line with other large British cities and to tackling problems which had been neglected for years. After this period of intensive activity, the reform impulse showed signs of weakening and the MOH ended up – out of necessity rather than choice – spending more time and effort making plans rather than implementing them. During the last two decades of the nineteenth century he collected, edited and analysed a vast amount of information on disease mortalities and sanitary conditions in the town. These findings were used not only to target more efficiently sanitary and health problems but also to fight complacency among city councillors and the public.[9]

In the collection and analysis of data, the MOH used the sixteen administrative wards into which Birmingham was divided in the 1880s.[10] This approach revealed sharply the wide variations in death rates between the run-down central quarters and suburban residential areas. In the 1890s, death rates in insanitary central wards such as St Mary's and St Bartholomew's (over 26 per 1,000 population) were almost twice as high as those experienced in the 'healthiest' wards such as Edgbaston (14 per 1,000 population). Furthermore, this approach enabled the MOH to contrast mortality with sanitary conditions in each ward.[11] Although Hill had come to accept that some diseases were caused by micro-organisms, he was a strong advocate of environmentalist sanitarianism until the end of his career in 1902. Thus, the fact that the death rates for the wards of St Mary's and St Bartholomew's were exceptionally high year after year was, in his opinion, the 'inevitable result of the conditions under which life has to be lived in them'.[12] Houses in these wards were clustered in courts, toilet facilities were the worst in the town, streets and yards were dirty and unpaved, and the atmosphere was polluted by factories and workshops.

---

[8]   A.S. Wohl, *Endangered Lives. Public Health in Victorian Britain* (London, 1984), pp. 179–82; E.P. Hennock, *Fit and Proper Persons. Ideal and Reality in Nineteenth-Century Urban Government* (London, 1973), pp. 111–16.
[9]   (BPRO) Birmingham Health Committee (HC), minutes 23. 7. 1901 item 6933; 10. 6. 1902 item 7478; 9. 12. 1902 item 7774; *Annual Reports of the Medical Officer of Health for Birmingham* (hereafter *Annual Report*) for 1872–1900 and in particular for 1874, pp. 15–17; for 1882, pp. 3–4; for 1885, pp. 57–67; for 1888, pp. 46–53; for 1897, pp. 6–10, 20–33; for 1898, pp. 8–15, 34–40. See also, A. Mayne, *The Imagined Slum. Newspaper Representation in Three Cities, 1870–1914* (Leicester, 1993), pp. 57–97.
[10]   For instance, *Annual Report for 1885*, pp. 57–67; R. Woods, 'Mortality and sanitary conditions in the "Best governed city in the world" – Birmingham, 1870 – 1910', *Journal of Historical Geography*, 4 (1978), 35–56.
[11]   *Annual Report for 1885*, pp. 57–67, for 1888, pp. 14–16, for 1897, pp. 9–10, 20–29, for 1898, pp. 8–15, 20–26, 34–9.
[12]   *Annual Report for 1898*, p. 8.

However, the major reason for high death rates in the central wards, the MOH argued, were back-to-back houses which had only front ventilation.

> [It had been a] very common practice in Birmingham to erect houses in rows back to back and in some cases this peculiarity of disposition is apparently necessary in order to prevent their falling or being blown down, so flimsily are they built; but such a mode of construction prevents what is of immense importance – a through draft.[13]

When the concerns of public health moved from cleaning up the environment to educating people in the early twentieth century, the notion of the unhealthy area maintained its significance as a major conceptual tool for defining urban health problems. The only difference was that Alfred Hill's successor, Dr John Robertson, did not attribute high mortality rates primarily to environmental problems. He argued that a very important reason why the inner-city wards experienced exceptionally high death rates was that their residents' attitudes and behaviour – social contacts, bodily maintenance, treatment of illnesses and diet – were 'unhealthy'.[14] New health care services, many of which were intrusive, were aimed at instilling 'the laws of health' in the people who lived in the central wards. For example, the first municipal health visitors worked almost exclusively in the unhealthy areas, visiting homes and advising mothers on domestic arrangements and infant care.[15]

In death rate tables these 'unhealthy' central wards were at the top, and in maps – in visual depictions of the problem – they were always shaded black as shown in Figure 8.2. By means of these charts and maps, which illustrated mortality rates in different wards or linked mortality rates with 'unhealthy' ways of life, complex and confusing urban health problems were given a simpler form. This simplification helped both public health experts and executives to target problems, but it also reinforced existing social relations. The division between the unhealthy, less unhealthy and healthy areas took a strong imaginative hold on people, serving to promote residential and social

---

13   *Annual Report for 1873*, p. 19; for 1898, pp. 8–15, 34–9. Mayne, 'The Imagined Slum', pp. 57–97.
14   *Special Report of the MOH on Infant Mortality in the City of Birmingham* (Birmingham: City of Birmingham, Health Department, 1904); *Report of the MOH on the Unhealthy Conditions in the Floodgate Street Area and the Municipal Wards of St Mary, St Stephen, and St Bartholomew* (Birmingham: City of Birmingham, Health Department, 1904); *Special Report by the MOH on Further Measures for the Prevention of Consumption in the City of Birmingham* (Birmingham: City of Birmingham, Health Department, 1906); *Annual Report for 1910*, pp. 13–15.
15   BPRO, HC, minutes 24. 7. 1900 item 6418; 9. 10. 1900 items 6469 & 6470; 14. 2. 1905 items 9115 and 9134; 14. 1. 1908 item 907; 19. 2. 1908 item 1001; 14. 4. 1908 item 1109.

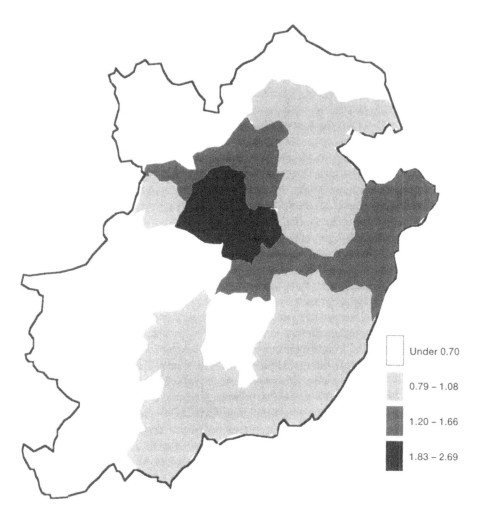

Figure 8.2: Death rates from pulmonary tuberculosis, Birmingham 1912.
By comparing the death rates in different wards, the Birmingham authorities
defined the 'unhealthy areas' and legitimated municipal intervention in them.

Source: *Annual report of the Medical Officer of Health for Birmingham, 1912.*

differentiation in the city. When the categorisations of this type become official, 'they become increasingly real'.[16]

The political assumptions which lay behind these allegedly neutral illustrations become clear when the Birmingham maps are compared with those produced in Gothenburg. For most of the nineteenth century, policy-makers in Gothenburg had been convinced that hospital beds would give better value than sanitary reforms and, accordingly, municipal health policy had essentially been oriented toward the individual. However, in the 1870s a number of environmental questions found a place on the agenda and sanitary reforms were carried through in the socially mixed inner-city wards. The vigour and pace of the reform slackened considerably when the same services were proposed for working-class areas on the outskirts of the town.[17] In the 1890s, the First City Physician for Gothenburg, Dr Henric Benckert, routinely compared death rates in these different wards, but he did not go on to analyse the differences in the same way as his Birmingham counterpart. Benckert reported that damp, filthy, ill-ventilated flats, the low standard of amenities such as water supply, drainage, privies and yards, and some wider environmental problems caused serious health problems in Gothenburg, but he did not link these insanitary conditions with any particular ward. Similarly, his successor, Dr Karl Gezelius, often argued that people's unhealthy habits made them susceptible to diseases, but he did not specify any ward where people's attitudes and behaviour would have been particularly 'irrational' and 'unhealthy'. Instead of defining insanitary areas, the Gothenburg authorities paid their attention to low-rent dwellings, which were scattered in the socially-mixed city centre and in working-class areas. Instead of defining the areas where, for example, the death rate from tuberculosis was high, they pinpointed the precise location of all houses where someone had died of tuberculosis as shown in Figure 8.3.[18] Individuals, not political boundaries, were the important criteria for creating the maps.

Similarly, the Gothenburg health authorities did not aim new health services at people who lived in problem areas, but at problem families or problem individuals irrespective of where they lived.[19] The Public Health Department

---

[16]   T.M. Porter, *Trust in Numbers. The Pursuit of Objectivity in Science and Public Life* (Princeton, 1995), p. 42.

[17]   M.C. Nelson and J. Rogers, 'Cleaning up the cities: Application of the first comprehensive public health law in Sweden', *Scandinavian Journal of History*, 19 (1994), 17–39; O. Wetterberg and G. Axelsson, *Smutsguld and dödligt hot. Renhållning och återvinning i Göteborg 1864–1930* (Gothenburg, 1995), pp. 97–169.

[18]   See, for example, *Göteborgs helsovårdsnämnds årsberättelser* (hereafter *Årsberättelse) för 1890–1920*; C. Lindman, *Sundhets- och befolkningsförhållanden i Sveriges städer 1851–1909* (Hälsingborg, 1909), pp. 66–95.

[19]   *GSH* 1908:252 and minutes 10. 12. 1908 item 18; 1909:197 and minutes 28. 10. 1909 item 5; *Årsberättelse för 1911*, pp. 8–13; *för 1912*, pp. 9–13.

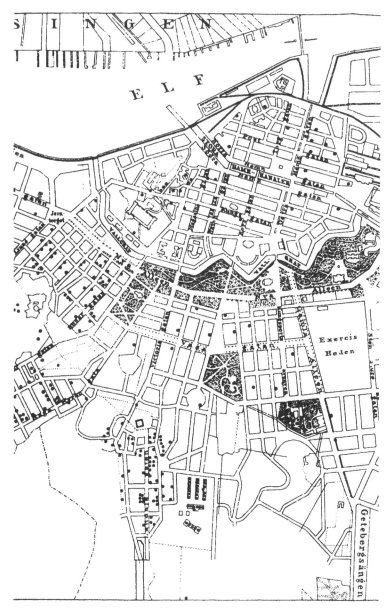

Figure 8.3: Deaths from tuberculosis in Gothenburg, 1904.
Instead of defining 'unhealthy areas', the Gothenburg authorities focused
their attention on individual homes.

Source: Göteborgs helsovårdsnämnds årsberättelser för1904.

did not employ health visitors who would have gone from door to door in the poorest wards, or infant welfare visitors who would have visited the homes of all newborn babies in working-class areas. They employed district nurses who visited the sick and two 'household consultants' who together visited about a hundred 'problem families' a year, spending on average four days with each family. The voluntary society, which launched the infant welfare campaign in association with municipal authorities, did not send nurses to the homes of all newborn babies but only to the homes where the mother was not able to breastfeed her child.[20]

At first glance, the different ways in which the Birmingham and Gothenburg authorities 'mapped' their towns do not raise any profound questions. In Birmingham, which in 1901 contained more than half a million people, the health authorities had good practical reasons to focus on 'unhealthy areas' and not to try to keep an eye on individuals. The Gothenburg authorities, by contrast, were able to deal with problem houses and problem families, since Gothenburg was still a relatively small city with a population of 140,000. However, the size of the population is not the sole, nor even the primary explanation for these differences. Health authorities in small British cities, such as Leicester, often chose the same approach as their counterparts in Birmingham, using the notion of the unhealthy area as a conceptual tool in analysing health problems.[21]

A crucial clue to explaining these different approaches lies in the political aspirations of urban élites. The analyses and illustrations of urban health problems were a vehicle for managing urban meaning and thus critical for the economic and political success of the élites.[22] In Birmingham and in many other British cities, where the development of socially segregated residential areas had been inseparably linked with the increasing political and economic power of the middle class, public health policy also reflected and reinforced the idea of segregation. Underlying the debate about public health problems was an assumption, sometimes made explicit, that towns were by their very nature socially segregated, and that the segregation in, for example, Birmingham was not clear enough. The MOH for Birmingham considered it regrettable that a large number of well-paid artisans, who could have lived in other residential

---

[20]   *GSH* 1909:252, 25–6; 1910:59; 1911:27; 1916:313, 1916:376; 1917:97 and minutes and discussion 19. 4. 1917 item 7; 1917:489 and minutes and discussion 10. 1. 1918 item 17; 1919:546 and minutes 22. 12. 1919 item 14. Göteborgs Stadsarkiv, Göteborgs Sjuksköterskebyrå, Ämnesordnande handlingar 1914–55, Redogörelser för kommunalsköterskornas verksamhet.

[21]   *Annual Report of the MOH for Leicester for 1903*, see Appendix, Special Diarrhoea Map; for 1910, see Appendix, Map of the Borough of Leicester Showing Municipal Wards, classed according to their average Mortality.

[22]   For discussion about urban meaning, see for example M. Savage and A. Warde, *Urban Sociology, Capitalism and Modernity* (London, 1993).

areas, put their health at risk by living in slum quarters.[23] While in Birmingham the political and social élite regulated the city from their enclaves outside the city centre, the Gothenburg upper middle class, a smaller and more closely-knit group, consolidated its power by living in the city centre or areas nearby. Contemporary reports give the impression that many municipal wards in Gothenburg had a fairly wide mix of social classes. The development of residential segregation was slow, in the eyes of contemporaries at least, and the poor and the well-to-do still lived relatively close to each other, especially in the centre of the city.[24] It is evident that a clear spatial separation of social groups did not have the same political and economic significance in Gothenburg as it had in Birmingham, and thus the notions of the unhealthy and healthy areas were not important conceptual tools in explaining urban health questions. Urban inequality was expressed spatially also in Gothenburg, but the relationship between the social classes and urban space was different from that in Birmingham. Thus, instead of classifying areas as 'good' and 'bad', the Gothenburg health authorities classified houses.

Regulating urban life

We now turn to a comparison of the anti-tuberculosis campaigns in Birmingham and Gothenburg, examining, first, the ways in which the rights and responsibilities of the healthy, the sick and the medical profession were defined in these campaigns and, second, the political implications of these definitions. In most British and Swedish cities, health authorities launched their anti-tuberculosis campaigns at the turn of the century. As a result of the discoveries of Robert Koch and other contemporary scientists, health authorities 'knew' that in the majority of cases, the tubercle bacillus was transmitted from person to person by droplet infection and that it depended on a newly infected person's level of resistance as to whether they developed the active disease or not. These new, apparently 'indisputable' facts, it was argued, equipped health authorities to tackle the problem by 'prescribing' the direction and form an effective anti-tuberculosis campaign was to take.[25]

---

[23]   *Report of the MOH on the Unhealthy Conditions* (Birmingham, 1904).

[24]   See, for example, Wallqvist, *Bostadsförhållandena*, pp. 4–11; Lindman, *Sundhets-och befolkningsförhållanden*, pp. 66–95; Variations in death rates between different wards were smaller in Gothenburg than in Birmingham. In Gothenburg, death rates for wards varied from 13 to 19 per 1,000 population in the 1890s, whereas in Birmingham they ranged between 14 and 26. See for instance, *Årsberättelse för 1892*, p. 46; *för 1898*, table 18.

[25]   *GSH 1903*:141; *Betänkande och förslag af den utaf Kungl. Maj:t den 20 Oktober tillsatta kommitté för verkställande af utredning angående åtgärder för människotuberkulosens bekämpande I* (Stockholm 1907); G. Dixon, *Lectures on the Prevention of Consumption Delivered to the Birmingham and Derbyshire Tuberculosis*

However, the new 'truth' about tuberculosis permitted widely different definitions of the disease and left ample room for disagreement on what measures would be the most appropriate and effective to tackle the problem. Some public health experts and executives concentrated their attention almost exclusively on the tubercle bacillus, seeking to create the impression that tuberculosis was a medical problem, devoid of deep social roots. For them, the campaign against tuberculosis was basically a scientific battle against the bacillus led by experts in medicine and public health. Others emphasised the importance of research findings indicating that the bacillus did not entirely explain the phenomenon of tubercular disease and that susceptibility also played a significant role. From this perspective, the problem could be approached as though tuberculosis was born and bred of unhealthy habits, which weakened the body's own defence mechanism and could be solved through health education. Yet others, albeit only a few, focused on social and environmental factors such as poverty and defective housing which were believed to make people susceptible to tuberculosis and other diseases. These health experts and executives called for changes in the economic and social structures of society. Health authorities in Birmingham and Gothenburg combined these approaches, fighting the bacterial, behavioural and environmental causes of diseases at the same time. They both had, however, a tendency to give weight to one line of reasoning and to play down the others, depending on their public health traditions and on wider political and social aims behind the health policy. All these approaches, albeit based on 'value-free' research findings, advanced particular political ideals and professional aspirations.

What public health authorities saw when they examined the problem of tuberculosis depended very much on what they expected or wanted to see. The Gothenburg health authorities saw unhygienic flats, attics and cellar dwellings. They viewed tuberculosis, first and foremost, as a 'dwelling-disease' (*bostadssjukdom*) which chose most of its victims from overcrowded, ill-ventilated, dark and filthy homes.[26] As proof of the link between defective housing and tuberculosis, health authorities cited investigations conducted in Sweden and abroad. In France, as in Sweden, housing problems were closely integrated into the medical and social understanding of tuberculosis. The Chief Tuberculosis Officer for Gothenburg, Dr Gösta Göthlin, often used French

---

Visitors (Derby c. 1910), p. 3; *Annual Report for 1898*, pp. 28–30; *for 1903*, p. 27; H. Sutherland, 'The extent of the disease and the sources of infection', in H. Sutherland (ed.), *The Control and Eradication of Tuberculosis: A Series of International Studies* (Edinburgh, 1911), pp. 5–23.
[26]   *GSH 1900*:104; 1902:2; 1908:252; *Årsberättelse för 1902*, p. 40; *för 1911*, pp. 10–13; *för 1912*, pp. 10–13; Göthlin, 'Några bostadshygieniska reformkrav', pp. 1152–6.

research to support his arguments.[27] There was also an abundance of evidence available from Germany, Britain and the United States which backed up the health authorities' conclusion: the worse the housing conditions the higher the death rate from tuberculosis. This certainly gave cause for concern, since in Gothenburg a large proportion of inhabitants lived in small and overcrowded flats. In 1910, about 63 per cent of the housing stock in Gothenburg had only one room, or one room and a kitchen, and 38 per cent of town-dwellers lived at a density of more than two persons per room.[28]

In considering the role housing conditions played in the pathogenesis of tuberculosis, the Gothenburg authorities invoked ideas of 'soil' and 'seed'. Defective housing was doubly to blame. First, poor housing conditions rendered the human soil receptive: living in damp, mouldy, ill-ventilated and filthy dwellings gradually diminished the body's capacity to fight the infection and thus paved the way for the active disease.[29] This question failed, however, to attract widespread interest, and the discussion was usually determinedly steered towards the second aspect, the seed. The risk of infection was considered to be high in insanitary, overcrowded flats. Not only were the tubercle bacilli transmitted easily from person to person when people lived huddled together in small rooms, bacilli were also believed to thrive in filth, darkness and stationary air. Insanitary dwellings, it was argued, were an ideal breeding ground for bacilli.[30] To emphasise the seriousness of the matter the Tuberculosis Officer pointed out in 1911 that this problem was not limited to the poorest of the poor. Once tuberculosis had taken hold of the wage-earner, even relatively well-to-do working-class families were likely to face a life of deprivation. In his statement to the City Council, the Tuberculosis Officer argued that tubercular patients and their families ended up in the worst flats

---

[27] For discussion about French or Swedish research findings, see for example, *GSH 1908*:252; 1913:337; *Årsberättelse för 1911*, pp. 10–13; *för 1912*, pp. 10–13; Göthlin, 'Några bostadshygieniska reformkrav', pp. 1153–4. For the French anti-tuberculosis campaign, see D. S. Barnes, *The Making of a Social Disease. Tuberculosis in Nineteenth-Century France* (Berkeley, 1995), pp. 112–37.

[28] *Statistisk årsbok för Göteborg 1925*, pp. 99, 103, 105; W. Göranson and G. Rosander, 'Vad siffrorna säga om Göteborgarens sätt att bo', *Katalog för Göteborgs stads bostadutställning 'Bo bättre'* (Gothenburg, 1936), pp. 25–41; A. Attman, *Göteborgs Stadsfullmäktige 1863–1962. I:1. Göteborg 1863–1913* (Gothenburg, 1963), pp. 278–9.

[29] *GSH 1908*:252. See also, G.H. von Koch, 'Bostadsfrågan', in G.H. von Koch (ed.), *Social Handbok* (Stockholm, 1908), pp. 79, 82.

[30] *Årsberättelse för 1911*, p. 13; *GSH 1913*:337, pp. 2–3; Göthlin, 'Några bostadhygieniska reformkrav', pp. 1152–3; E. Almquist, *Allmän hälsovårdslära med särskildt afseende på svenska förhållanden för läkare, medicine studerande, hälsovårdsmyndigheter, tekniker m. fl.* (Stockholm, 1897), pp. 740–43; *idem, Hälsovårdslärans framsteg under senaste åren* (Stockholm, 1902), pp. 26–7; B. Buhre, 'Tuberkulosens bekämpande', in G. H. von Koch (ed.) *Social Handbok* (Stockholm, 1908), pp. 325–32.

and houses available as certainly as though 'a natural law' had forced them there.[31]

This definition of tuberculosis could have suggested a broad social reform movement, advocating wide-ranging measures to improve living and working conditions. Indeed, both the First City Physician and the Tuberculosis Officer argued vehemently that the problem could not be solved without more active municipal intervention in the housing market. The municipality should control private building and rental sectors, support co-operative enterprises, but it should also build houses. The Tuberculosis Officer pointed out that the social hygiene housing study, which was conducted in Gothenburg in 1911, had revealed that inhabitants were not solely to blame. In his opinion, the problem revolved around two cores: the conservatism of poor town-dwellers and the conservatism of decision-makers. While the former were unwilling to abandon their unhygienic habits, the latter adhered to their traditional views on how social problems should be tackled.[32]

The majority of city councillors in Gothenburg disagreed with these health officials, insisting that a housing reform must be left to the market place.[33] Thus, in order to secure City Council's backing to the municipal tuberculosis scheme, the health officials had to adapt the definition of the problem to this majority view. The problem of tuberculosis was to be alleviated, at least in the short term, by removing tubercular patients who lived in small insanitary flats to hospitals. This view was a kind of compromise: while it included a tacit admission that the housing situation was extremely difficult, it also gave the City Council an excuse to postpone a serious discussion about the housing problem. Moreover, in the eyes of many policy-makers, hospitalisation successfully interwove the collective and individual good. While the healthy members of society were protected against the killer disease, tubercular patients were provided with the treatment they needed during the last months of their lives. Death in hospital was increasingly associated with positive

---

[31]   *GSH 1913*:337.

[32]   *GSH 1908*:252; 1909:197 and minutes 28. 10. 1909 item 5, 1911:216, pp. 12–13; 1913:337; Göthlin, 'Några bostadshygieniska reformkrav'. See also *GSH 1903*:122C, nr 15; Almquist, *Hälsovårdlärans framsteg*, pp. 26–7.

[33]   During the housing crisis in the late 1910s and early 1920s, municipal intervention was still vigorously opposed. However, in the 1920s, the municipality took a more active approach to the problem. See, for example, GSH 1917:14; 1923:113 and minutes and discussion 5. 4. 1923 item 13. Göthlin, 'Några bostadshygieniska reformkrav'; *Statens Offentliga Utredningar 1935:2: Betänkande och förslag rörande lån och årliga bidrag av statsmedel för främjande av bostadsförsörjning för mindre bemedlade barnrika familjer*, appendix 1, pp. 11–14.

values and qualities. Not only was it humane, hygienic and efficient, it was also well managed.[34]

Even though the First City Physician and the Tuberculosis Officer always stressed that medical care should be supplemented with other measures such as housing reform and health education, they, among other medical doctors, argued strongly for the hospitalisation of both early and advanced cases of tuberculosis. The medical profession in Sweden was usually all in favour of expanding publicly-funded medical care, since the majority of medical practitioners, including the medical élite, worked in the public sector.[35] The Gothenburg anti-tuberculosis campaign shows clearly that they were successful in shaping the definitions of health problems in ways which suited their professional aspirations. Gothenburg's first tuberculosis hospital was opened in 1903, and in 1914 health authorities provided 106 hospital and sanatorium beds for every 100 deaths from tuberculosis. Markedly fewer beds were available in Birmingham, where municipal and Poor Law authorities together provided only 57 hospital beds for every 100 deaths from tuberculosis.[36] What also illustrates the special emphasis which the Gothenburg authorities placed on the medical approach is their interest in the BCG-vaccine. The Gothenburg authorities started vaccine trials as early as 1927, whereas the Birmingham authorities and British authorities in general did not introduce the vaccine until the 1950s.[37] In Gothenburg, the anti-tuberculosis campaign was primarily a battle against the tubercle bacillus. Measures aimed at instructing people in healthy ways of life or at tackling environmental problems were secondary.

In Birmingham, and in Britain in general, public health doctors did not enjoy the same status as their counterparts in Gothenburg. Thus, compared with the Gothenburg public health programmes, the Birmingham campaigns reflected less the professional interests of public health doctors and more the interests of other important groups. As a result, the anti-tuberculosis campaign in Birmingham was an ambitious plan to regulate and organise the life of the

---

[34]   *GSH 1902*:90; 1903:122C nr 17, 1910:105; *Årsberättelse för 1904*, 34–5, för 1906, 42–4. See also, P. Ariès, *Western Attitudes Toward Death from the Middle Ages to the Present* (London, 1994), pp. 88–9.

[35]   G. Kearns, W.R. Lee and J. Rogers, 'The interaction of political and economic factors in the management of urban public health', in M.C. Nelson and J. Rogers (eds), *Urbanisation and the Epidemiological Transition* (Uppsala, 1989), pp. 9–81; E. Riska, 'The medical profession in the Nordic countries', in F.W. Hafferty and J. McKinlay (eds), *The Changing Medical Profession: An International Perspective* (New York, 1993), pp. 150–61; H. Bergstrand, 'Läkarekåren och provinsialläkareväsendet', in W. Kock (ed.), *Medicinalväsendet i Sverige 1813–1962* (Stockholm, 1963), pp. 107–57.

[36]   *Årsberättelse för 1913*, p. 9; *Annual Report for 1916*, p. 22.

[37]   A. Wallgren, 'Value of Calmette vaccination in prevention of tuberculosis in childhood', *Journal of American Medical Association*, 103 (1934), 1341–5; H. Anderson and H. Belfrage. 'Ten years experience of B.C.G.-vaccination at Gothenburg', *Acta Pædiatrica* 26 (1939), 1–11.

city. Instead of defining tuberculosis primarily as a medical problem and pinning their hopes on the isolation of infectious tubercular patients and on the vaccination of the healthy, authorities in Birmingham stressed the role of unhealthy attitudes and behaviour in causing tuberculosis.

To legitimate their definition of the problem, the Birmingham authorities made use of the same scientific findings as their Gothenburg counterparts: overcrowding, lack of sunshine and fresh air, want of cleanliness and malnourishment contributing to the high incidence of tuberculosis. However, they put a very different interpretation on these results. In general, what was considered to be dangerous was, as Michael Worboys has pointed out, certain kinds of social contact, with certain classes, in certain environments.[38] The Birmingham health campaigns stressed that tuberculosis was ubiquitous in these 'suspicious' situations. The disease was not only spreading in the homes where poor tubercular patients lived, but the danger was also lurking in any public space – in streets, tramcars, train compartments and public houses – where careless patients had been spitting and coughing. The germs of consumption lived in fine dust, 'which the slightest breath of air, the foot of a passer-by, the whisk of a lady's skirt, or a crawling infant distributes broadcast to be drawn into the lungs of all who are unfortunate enough to come in contact with it'.[39] Second, as tuberculosis was highly contagious, anyone could contract it and everyone was potentially ill. Tubercular patients who did not take precautions, the argument went, infected other people 'as certainly as one smallpox patient spreads the disease to those who come in contact with him'.[40]

The Birmingham authorities argued that people suffering from tuberculosis were, to an extent, responsible for contracting and developing the disease. The MOH, Dr John Robertson, pointed out that in the preceding decades the Birmingham Public Health Department had done much to reduce the number of susceptible people by improving housing and working conditions, by tackling wider environmental problems and by checking the quality of food.[41] What had largely been missing, he claimed, was a change in people's attitudes, values and behaviour. Instead of keeping themselves 'in such a condition of health as will enable them to resist the invasion of the germ', people increased their susceptibility to the infection by their unhealthy ways of life.[42]

Drinking in pubs and bad workshop conditions were regarded as major causes of the spread of tuberculosis. These factors were considered to both

---

[38] Worboys, 'The sanatorium treatment', p. 55.

[39] Dixon, *Lectures on the Prevention of Consumption*, pp. 4–5.

[40] *Special Report by the MOH on Further Measures for the Prevention of Consumption*, pp. 8–9.

[41] *Annual Report for 1903*, p. 27.

[42] *Special Report by the MOH on the Further Measures for the Prevention of Consumption*, p. 9.

render human 'soil' hospitable to infected 'seeds' and increase the number of 'seeds' to which individuals were exposed. First, by working in ill-ventilated, dark and damp factories and by 'soak(ing) themselves with drink every day' people weakened their resistance to infection. Second, in both workshops, where people worked in cramped conditions, and in pubs, where they coughed over one another and shared glasses, the risk of infection was believed to be extremely high.[43] Indeed, the MOH argued that drinking combined with ignorance and carelessness probably played a more important part than bad housing and poverty in causing tuberculosis and many other illnesses.[44]

Ironically, people also spent too much time in their ill-ventilated homes. '(B)y having an abundance of fresh air, which even in the centre of the city costs nothing and is of good quality' they could have, to a very large extent, prevented tuberculosis, claimed the MOH in his report in 1912.[45] Yet he never elaborated on the fortifying properties of 'fresh air', let alone the ways in which these properties would have assisted the body's defence mechanism in fighting against tuberculosis. Nor did he make any attempt to prove that the air in the city centre was of good quality. A more analytical approach was taken by the Medical Officer of the General Dispensary, Dr A. Carver, who argued that bad marketing and ignorance of food values paved the way to full-blown tuberculosis in many working-class families in Birmingham. By comparing the weekly diets of forty 'healthy' families and of forty families in which one or more persons suffered from tuberculosis, he was able to show that tuberculous families did not have as nutritious a diet as healthy families with the same level of income. Tuberculous families, he concluded, had spent their money on expensive articles such as beef instead of buying cheap nutritious food and, in consequence, both the overall energy value and the carbohydrate and fat content of their diet had been too low to protect them from tuberculosis. However, the value of his research finding was diminished by the fact that his conclusion was based on rather small groups of families and, more importantly, that these families were not chosen at random.[46]

In his study, Carver also paid attention to the question of housing. He praised the fact that, in most cases, people in Birmingham moved into better

---

[43]   *Report of the MOH on the Unhealthy Conditions*, pp. 17–18; *Annual Report for 1906*, pp. 62–3; *for 1912*, pp. 44–5; *Special Report by the MOH on the Further Measures for the Prevention of Consumption*, pp. 5–7.

[44]   *Report of the MOH on the Unhealthy Conditions*, pp. 17–18.

[45]   *Annual Report for 1912*, p. 6.

[46]   A.E. Carver, *An Investigation into the Dietary of the Labouring Classes of Birmingham, with Special Reference to its Bearing upon Tuberculosis* (Birmingham, 1914). Carver was not alone in thinking that the ignorance of nutritional values of different foodstuffs and bad marketing contributed to the prevalence of ill-health. See, for instance, D. E. Lindsay, *Report upon a Study on the Diet of the Labouring Classes in the City of Glasgow* (Glasgow, 1912), pp. 28–32; D.N. Paton, 'Introduction' in the above mentioned Report, p. 5.

houses and better neighbourhoods when their incomes rose. 'There is none of that clinging to a particular locality, which is so noticeable in the Londoner', he argued.[47] The MOH was more pessimistic. In his opinion, many people were used to their insanitary homes and did not actively seek better homes and better surroundings. Also, they worked in unhealthy environments, although working conditions were 'more or less under the control of the individual. If he thinks his workplace or the character of the work is likely to affect his health he has a remedy in his own hands by leaving the work'.[48] Tuberculosis, the argument went, was a disease born of ignorance, lack of initiative and will-power, and lack of self-control.

The answer to the problem was education. While voluntary societies enlightened the public as to how to keep in good health, the Birmingham health authorities concentrated on advising and 'reforming' tubercular patients whose disease was still 'curable'. The aim was to instil in patients and their families instincts of rational self-control and to inspire them to preserve their health by resisting 'unhealthy' habits, 'unhealthy' social contacts and 'unhealthy' environments. While in Gothenburg control measures were allied to medical paternalism, in Birmingham they were allied to an emphasis on individual responsibility. Individuals were expected to triumph over circumstances.

Conclusion

Owing to close international links between health officials, there were many universal features in Swedish and British public health campaigns. Yet these campaigns had also national and local characteristics which distinguished them from each other, and which clearly reveal the important role that political and otherwise legitimate social concerns played in determining the direction of health policy. Furthermore, national and local features illuminate the power of science as a legitimising rhetoric in policy-making. Many political and social aims, which would have been difficult to achieve via the electorate, were achieved through scientific, allegedly 'neutral' policies and procedures.

The ways in which the Birmingham and Gothenburg authorities analysed and illustrated health problems were affected by prevailing views on how urban society was organised. No matter how rigorously health officials conducted their statistical analyses, the questions they asked, the categories they used and the conclusions they drew were shaped by these political ideals. Thus, statistical tables, charts and maps which health officials produced always spoke of matters beyond their explicit content, constructing authoritative

---

[47]   Carver, *An Investigation*, p. 21.
[48]   *Birmingham Annual Report for 1924*, p. 29.

visions of the town and townspeople. In both Birmingham and Gothenburg, maps and charts which illustrated health problems legitimated the existing relationship between the social classes and urban space and thus served to ensure the reproduction of social structures which appealed to the urban élite.

Early twentieth-century public health campaigns against tuberculosis, infant mortality and venereal diseases played an important role in mediating urban conflicts and in regulating the life of the city. In both Birmingham and Gothenburg, the problem of tuberculosis was defined in a way which made environmental reforms appear inefficient and non-scientific. The work of Robert Koch and other contemporary scientists, which did not intrinsically force health authorities to jettison environmentalism, were determinedly reformulated in terms that provided a scientific foundation for measures aimed at the individual rather than wide-ranging sanitary reforms. The individualistic model of public health care enabled public health experts and executives to improve the health of the population and to regulate the life of cities without dealing directly with politically-charged environmental problems such as defective housing and unhealthy working conditions, or with the problem of poverty.

However, the individualistic models which the Birmingham and Gothenburg authorities chose were different. In Birmingham, the anti-tuberculosis campaign reflected and reinforced the ethos of individual responsibility. By adopting healthier, rational attitudes and behaviour, people would preserve their own health, but they would also contribute to the management of environmental problems. If people actively sought for better homes and surroundings, insanitary houses near polluting factories and workshops would become difficult to let. If individual workers tried to avoid unhealthy working conditions, offensive trades would find it impossible to attract a workforce. In Gothenburg, where the medical profession was influential in directing the policy, public health problems were medicalised and treated as conditions of individual bodies. Health authorities concentrated primarily on isolating and hospitalising people who suffered from tuberculosis and on keeping the healthy – and in particular children – out of the way of tubercle bacilli. Both approaches were justified by appeals to the authority of 'value-free' science and medicine.

Acknowledgement

I would like to thank Richard Rodger, Lucy Faire, Sally Horrocks and the editors for their helpful comments on an earlier version of this chapter.

9

Choices for town councillors in nineteenth-century Britain: investment in public heath and its impact on mortality

Robert Millward and Frances Bell

By the second half of the nineteenth century, legislation had firmly established that responsibility for policing the public's health was the legal obligation of local government. Elected town councillors in British industrial towns faced tremendous challenges and difficult choices in the course of fulfilling their responsibilities. The legacy of previous decades, in which rapid urban growth had gone largely unaccompanied by appropriate levels of planning and regulation, was the widespread pollution of the public environment. The antidote to the squalor, disease and high mortality, which was common in industrial towns, emerged as a tripart programme of prevention. It involved recognition of the need for invasive regulation of the public and private behaviour and property of citizens, for integrated and universal systems of waste removal and water supply and for the centralised local administration of the public's health. All were more or less novel concepts in the context of early nineteenth-century Britain and the process of their acceptance was long and fraught. It was arrived at by different paths, at different times and by varying degrees in different localities as both inhabitants and their elected representatives struggled towards an acceptance of new inroads into their private lives as citizens and into their pockets as ratepayers.

Whilst faltering at first, recognition of the necessity for radical actions became increasingly universal during the second half of the nineteenth century. However, precise plans for the required remedial and preventative works remained to be formulated locally. Whilst legislation was empowering, it was also initially permissive and failed to lay down the exact form of schemes to be adopted. The elected officials whose role it was to implement local 'rescue plans' worked within contemporary legal, financial and practical frameworks with numerous constraints. Local councils were composed largely of laymen who lacked knowledge of the fledgling technology of civil engineering and were ill-prepared to measure the merits of competing schemes and systems. Some councils, like Liverpool, responded by appointing Medical Officers of Health early in the 1840s and 1850s and were privy to qualified medical opinion on the methods of disease prevention. Others sought 'expert' advice from within the unfamiliar fields of environmental science and civil engineering and were largely at the mercy of their paid advisors during the planning and implementation of reform programmes.

The avenues open to local government in terms of financing hugely expensive clean-up campaigns varied according to the existence of civic assets in property and trading and the size of local tax bases. If they lacked a source of special revenue such as Doncaster racecourse or Southend pier and were unfortunate in failing to encompass affluent suburbs, local councils who spent on public health projects were almost inevitably required to tighten their purse-strings in other areas such as education and policing. The alternative was to increase taxes on residents in the form of higher rates. The second half of the nineteenth century witnessed a complex interplay between a hostile disease environment, a set of largely untried social and technical instruments in the form of new sanitation technologies and monitoring systems and, thirdly, painful economic choices in the allocation of resources for health improvements. Central government's minimal intervention in local public health issues also helped to ensure that policy and planning was shaped by local characteristics and circumstances, that is, by the priorities and ingenuity of local officials and their paid advisors and by the response of inhabitants to the decisions made by their elected representatives.

The result of local autonomy in the public health sphere was diversity. Responses to public health issues varied according to the nature and degree of problems faced by local authorities and the availability of resources to counteract them. In these circumstances, a national picture of urban local government's conduct in response to public health 'crisis' is difficult to paint. Case-studies of towns based on the minutes of council meetings such as those by Hennock for Birmingham and the Pooleys for Manchester have considerably enhanced our understanding of the contemporary debates.[1] As Szreter has pointed out, however, the coverage of existing studies of individual towns and

---

[1]		E.P. Hennock, *Fit and Proper Persons: Ideal and Reality in Nineteenth Century Government* (London, 1973); M.E. Pooley and C.G. Pooley, 'Health, Society and Environment in Victorian Manchester', in R.I. Woods and J.H. Woodward (eds), *Urban Disease and Mortality in the 19th Century*, (London, 1984), pp. 148–75.

regions remains slight at present with comprehensive coverage some considerable time away.[2]

A complementary method for understanding and analysing the response of local government to the problems of urban public health is available via an alternative route. Local taxation returns provide information on the spending records of all town councils in England and Wales from 1870 and are detailed in the information they provide about public health spending. From the information we have on the outcomes of their decisions it is possible to infer and deduce something of the behaviour of town councillors. When the timing and scale of spending on public health is related to levels of mortality from the Registrar-General's returns it becomes possible to measure the extent of local government's success in countering the growing urban problems faced by their communities.

In examining the spending patterns of local councils we are concerned with two main issues. First, how much attention was actually given to solving public health problems? Can we quantify the size of the public health effort and was it a larger or smaller activity than policing, education, tramways, gas or electricity? Second, how effective was the public health effort at tackling contemporary problems and, specifically, can the differences in spending across towns or over time be linked to changing levels of mortality? These questions require new approaches and the methods we propose to use here include an explicit recognition of the role of economic forces in the decisions of town councillors.

Decisions and outcomes for capital works programmes

The second half of the nineteenth century witnessed a massive expansion of the infrastructure serving Britain. Railways were a key element rapidly connecting all parts of the country whilst there was a mushrooming of waterworks, roads, workhouses, trams, hospitals, electricity stations and gasworks in urban areas. Although private gas companies, charity hospitals and private landowners' water supplies contributed to the growth of the urban infrastructure, it was overwhelmingly a public sector initiative and one in which local government was dominant. From the 1850s, local authorities carried out over 90 per cent of *all* government investment. By the early 1900s, this was nearly as large as the capital expenditure of the whole of manufacturing industry. How local authorities coped with these spending programmes given their continued reliance on a fairly narrow

---

[2]   S. Szreter, 'The Importance of Social Intervention in Britain's Mortality Decline c. 1850–1914: A Reinterpretation of the Role of Public Health', *Social History of Medicine*, 1 (1988), 1–37.

tax base – the local rates – had not been analysed in any detail prior to the recent work at Manchester on the hitherto untapped detail in the Local Taxation Returns.[3] The latter have proved a very rich data source for revealing the pattern of spending and finance of different local authority types in different regions. It is clear that urban areas suffered from massively diminishing returns as population increases generated disproportionate demands for spending on the infrastructure. In the absence of a local land, profit or sales tax, the burden fell on the property tax leading to 'rates revolts' and to town councils venturing into property and trading activities to generate new income sources.

The significance of public health reform within this general pattern of spending is an issue that has received little attention to date. The traditional literature on public health focused on its legislative and administrative history and often on the personalities, like Chadwick and Simon, surrounding central government initiatives. But reform programmes were all financed and executed by local government. Szreter's recent research on mortality includes the speculation that, for both airborne and water-borne diseases, public health reform programmes were just as important as the rising living standards and better diets stressed by McKeown.[4] Szreter was able to quote only broad aggregates of local authority spending, however, as the quantitative magnitude of expenditure on public health and its phasing over time and dispersion across towns and regions had not then been comprehensively set out.[5] Williamson, at the end of *Coping with City Growth*, admits that the information for assessing the impact of sanitation investment is not yet available and, *a fortiori*, that there is as yet no estimate of the size of different kinds of sanitary investment and their separate quantitative impacts on mortality.[6] Even Brown, who has tried more than most to make international comparisons in this area, has found UK data more scanty than that for the USA and Germany.[7]

---

[3]   R. Millward and S. Sheard, 'The Urban Fiscal Problem 1870–1914: Government Expenditure and Finances in England and Wales', *Economic History Review*, 48 (1995), 501–35.

[4]   Szreter, 'The Importance of Social Intervention in Britain's Mortality Decline'; T. McKeown and R.G. Record, 'Reasons for the Decline of Mortality in England and Wales during the 19th Century', *Population Studies*, 16 (1962), 94–122; T. McKeown, R.G. Brown and R. Record, 'An Interpretation of the Modern Rise in Population in Europe', *Population Studies*, 26 (1972), 345–82.

[5]   But see R. Millward and F. Bell, 'Economic Factors in the Decline of Mortality in Late Nineteenth century Britain', *European Review of Economic History*, 2 (1998), pp. 263–88.

[6]   J.G. Williamson, *Coping with City Growth During the British Industrial Revolution* (Cambridge, 1990) pp. 286, 290.

[7]   J. Brown, 'Who Paid for the Sanitary City?: Issues and Evidence ca. 1910', paper presented to session C7, Eleventh International Economic History Conference, Milan, 1994.

Activities which one might class as public health range very widely, from inspection of premises, construction of sewers and street scavenging, to monitoring of milk supplies, disseminating good childbirth practices and controlling factory effluent to rivers. Some of these activities were being provided 'collectively' by Improvement Commissioners or municipal boroughs from the early eighteenth century.[8] As Razzell has argued, they may have contributed to the late eighteenth-century decline in mortality.[9] Public provision on a large scale can be dated from the middle of the nineteenth century and we can use data in the Local Taxation Returns on the spending patterns of local authorities as a measure of contemporary commitment to public health. Of course, expenditure data is at best a measure of the 'input' into health services rather than of its effectiveness and it does not cover the private sector, both of which qualifications are relevant to our conclusions.

Public health was a very capital intensive activity in the nineteenth century as the infrastructure of sewers, waterworks and streets was laid down. The large capital outlays for the construction programmes were often financed by loans and stock issues which generated a stream of annual loan charges (interest payments and repayment of principal) to set alongside the annual labour, fuel and other items of recurrent expenditure. It was the total of current expenditure plus annual loan charges, which had to be financed by the rates. Mitchell's data provide a national perspective on spending and suggest that average capital expenditure on sewers, refuse disposal, baths, commons, parks and hospitals averaged £1.5 million per annum for all local authorities in England and Wales in the 1880s.[10] Public health therefore accounted for approximately one-fifth of all local authority capital expenditure on services (that is, excluding markets, gasworks, property and other trading activities). A portion of expenditures on water resource programmes should be added to the public health figure since piped water supplies clearly performed a health-preserving function. Unfortunately the industrial usage of water cannot be separately identified from its public and domestic use. The average figure for capital investment in water was £1.5 million per annum in the 1880s. Adding this to the separate public health figure, we arrive at a (perhaps inflated) estimate of the public health effort averaging two-fifths of total local authority capital expenditure on services. Turning to current expenditure, the proportion of total expenditure dedicated to public health functions is even smaller. In the 1880s the annual labour, fuel, staffing and other operating costs of refuse disposal, baths, commons, parks, sewers and hospitals

---

[8]   E.L. Jones and M.E. Falkus, 'Urban Improvements and the English Economy in the 17th and 18th centuries', in P. Borsay (ed.), *The 18th Century English Town* (London, 1990).

[9]   P.E. Razzell, 'An Interpretation of the Modern Rise of Population: A Critique', *Population Studies*, 28 (1974), 5–17.

[10]   B.R. Mitchell , *British Historical Statistics* (Cambridge, 1988).

averaged no more than about £1.25 million for all the local authorities in England and Wales.[11] This was small beer next to the £3.4 million spent on police and £21.4 million on other services, even when trading is excluded. However, these 'other services' include street cleansing and scavenging, lighting and a wide range of public works with health dimensions which are not easy to separate and quantify as part of public health expenditure from the above secondary sources.

In order to obtain a clearer picture of the items on which town councils were spending, we have looked in detail at information in the Local Taxation Returns on a sample of thirty-six towns. These were selected to provide a good geographic coverage of England and Wales and to include towns with wide-ranging characteristics. The sample includes towns whose staple industries have particular working conditions such as textiles, mining and glass. Ports and seaside towns located in ameliorating proximity to the sea for waste disposal purposes are also represented, as are small rural towns like Great Torrington and Thetford whose small populations and limited health problems throw conditions in the large industrial towns of the North and Midlands into sharper relief. A full list of the thirty-six towns including mortality rates and population densities in 1871 is given in Table 9.1.

Close inspection of the Local Taxation Returns confirms that all categories in the 'sanitary' account of each town were public health items, including expenditure on scavenging, street repair, flood channels, slaughterhouses, parks, other open spaces and refuse destructors as well as sewers, baths, water supplies and hospitals.[12] Table 9.2 shows the extent of local government spending on some of these different elements during the period 1906–13. Capital expenditure on sewers accounted for about 8 per cent of all local authority investment or 12 per cent if trading activities are excluded. Adding in expenditure on streets and related public works suggests that total sanitation investment was actually of the order of £27,021 per town or 46 per cent of the total. Finally, if water supply is included, we arrive at a sum of £44,522 per annum, which is three-quarters of all local authority non-trading investment – a share that held for most of the post-1870 period. Even if one were to discount some of the investment in water supply and roads as being driven by narrow transport and industrial demands, the remaining investment in public health accounted for a major share of total local authority capital expenditure. Public health expenditure clearly played a significant role in determining the overall shape of local authority spending

    [11]   Mitchell, *British Historical Statistics*; Millward and Sheard, 'The Urban Fiscal Problem 1870–1914', 529.
    [12]   See F. Bell and R. Millward , 'Public Health Expenditures and Mortality in England and Wales 1870–1914', *Continuity and Change*, 13 (1998) 221–49 for more detail.

Table 9.1: Mortality, housing and population in a sample of 36 towns in England and Wales in 1871 (based on registration districts)

Town	Deaths per 000 population	Population	Persons per acre	Houses per acre
Liverpool	38.709	241240	97.666	31.179
Bristol	31.451	63178	83.679	35.872
Northampton	31.300	49393	2.4362	.36439
Manchester	30.978	254470	19.584	4.9907
Leeds	29.979	159580	11.601	3.9666
Swansea	29.345	56057	1.2692	.20013
Leicester	28.074	92507	28.908	5.9412
Preston	27.813	114520	1.6956	.24011
Norwich	27.737	79640	10.658	2.4329
Carlisle	26.588	39416	.56989	.08688
Bradford	26.383	252330	6.0640	.68277
Nottingham	25.942	82840	41.503	8.9734
Oxford	25.133	20929	7.1430	2.0730
Marlborough	24.273	10011	.24291	.01545
St Helens	24.161	44121	4.8373	.84541
Wrexham	23.961	48204	.73643	.02436
York	23.712	63724	.77199	.10811
Tottenham	22.913	20512	4.4188	.79642
Plymouth	22.619	68262	45.783	4.8518
Doncaster	22.350	44341	.39129	.03553
Wolverhampton	22.203	135110	2.4611	.23857
Southampton	22.171	47043	35.531	6.7598
Gt Torrington	21.837	1486	.20265	.00892
Luton	21.040	33746	.82638	.07775
Sunderland	20.660	109970	9.5651	1.0811
Hastings	20.471	34194	2.4377	.29657
Carmarthen	20.430	35683	.20699	.01148
Kingston	19.957	53816	2.1524	.10227
Hanley	19.927	20876	4.2578	1.5109
Lincoln	19.738	51068	.32160	.03349
Thetford	19.172	18151	.15034	.00757
Shaftesbury	18.735	13184	.36127	.01334
Louth	18.051	34902	.20445	.01459
Ramsgate	17.649	23458	2.8968	.32872
Richmond	16.439	13565	.16726	.01120

Sources: Registrar-General's Annual Reports and Censuses of Population

**Table 9.2: The public health share of local authority investment
(average annual capital expenditure 1906–13 per sample town in £'000)**

Sewers	6955
Streets	10008
Other sanitation	10058
Water supply	17500
Total sanitation and water	44522
Education, police and other non-trading	
services	14199
Total services	**58721**
Trading activities	25999
Total	**84721**

Notes: Sources are annual Local Taxation Returns 1905/6 to 1912/13. Data refers to financial years ending in the year quoted.

patterns and appears to have been at the root of many of the financial strains experienced.

The wealth of a local authority would clearly affect how far and with what intensity it could extend its public health effort. How did the pattern of local authority spending on public health change in the course of the half-century up to the First World War, and for what reasons? Aggregate local authority investment showed a massive peak at the end of the nineteenth century.[13] To some extent this peak reflected the new technology and huge expansion in electricity and tramways. But it is now clear that expenditures on water supply and sanitation also underwent large increases in the 1890s and early 1900s, as is illustrated in Figure 9.1. Expenditure on different elements of public health provision differed considerably in timing and scale. Figure 9.1 shows that in the early part of our period (and separate estimates suggest this can include the 1870s) investment in water supply was running at more than three times the level of investment in sewers. This was not without its own unfavourable side effects as flood channels, sewers and other drainage channels were initially overstretched by the enhanced water supplies. By the 1890s, sewer investment

---

[13]   J. Wilson, 'The Finance of Municipal Capital Expenditure in England and Wales, 1870–1914', *Financial History Review*, 4 (1997), 31–50; Millward and Sheard, 'The Urban Fiscal Problem 1870–1914'.

was approaching 60 per cent of the level of water as drainage systems were being planned and constructed to cope with the now more ample local supplies of water.

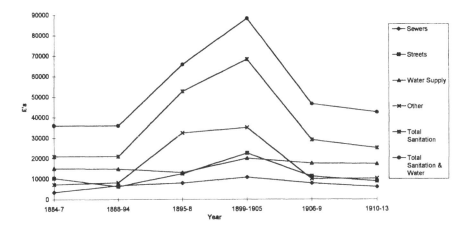

Figure 9.1: Capital expenditure out of loans for sanitation and water supply in 36 towns in England and Wales 1884–1913

Source: Annual Local Taxation Returns for England and Wales 1884–1914.
Notes: Data relate to the financial year ending in the year in question. There are thirty-six observations each year excepting Blackpool in 1901 and Tottenham in 1902.

Szreter has highlighted the discrepancy in timing that exists between the period commonly believed to mark the zenith of public health activity in Britain (associated with individuals such as Chadwick and Simon), and the date at which mortality levels actually began to comprehensively decline. Public health policy achieved its desired outcome of producing viable public utilities only through a lengthy process of local planning and decision-making. To forget this process is to entirely misjudge the timescale of reform. Local government expenditure data demonstrates that peak investment in sanitary facilities was firmly confined to the end of the nineteenth century rather than to its middle decades. Whilst peak public health spending clearly post-dated the limited mortality decline beginning in the 1870s it was entirely coincident with the period in which mortality decline was comprehensive across all ages, sexes and disease groups.[14]

What factors account for the apparent delay in town council commitment to public health improvements? Why was it not until the 1890s that councillors were prepared to invest substantially in sewer and street improvements? One factor of which town councillors were painfully aware was that sanitation issues could not be contained within their own jurisdictional boundaries. What Bolton mills poured into the Irwell affected the residents of Salford.[15] Not until the late twentieth century were River Authorities in Britain given strong powers and made the central focus for the development of water supplies and sewer systems. In the meantime, procedures for reconciling the needs of the likes of Bolton and Salford had to rely on joint consultative committees or, as in the case of Manchester, on one local authority expanding its boundaries to embrace the whole of a naturally occurring drainage district.

There was a financial predicament which councillors faced from the very beginning of each capital works programme, namely the need to raise loans to allow the construction of water and sewer systems and street improvements. In the early part of the century local authorities had little financial credibility; some were rotten boroughs and most lacked a proper constitutional base for electing representatives from the ratepaying population. This as much as anything explains why demand for the expansion of water supplies in the first decades of the century was met by the private sector in the form of new joint-stock companies.[16] The 1834 Municipal Corporations Act provided the constitutional base for ratepayer representation and this was exploited by a wave of new municipal boroughs in the Midlands and the north of England. Even at mid-century, councils lacked autonomous powers for raising funds through mortgage loans and in order to raise finance had generally to resort to applying for a special Act of Parliament. It was a private Act of 1869 which gave powers to the Metropolitan Board of Works to raise stock of £2.6 million. This was followed in the 1870s by Acts for other large towns including Manchester, Leeds, Birmingham, Leicester and Liverpool.[17] In fact, since they

---

[14]   R.I. Woods, 'Mortality Patterns in the Nineteenth Century', in R.I. Woods and J.H. Woodward (eds), *Urban Disease and Mortality in the 19th Century* (London, 1984), pp. 37–64.

[15]   See also Hennock, *Fit and Proper Persons* for Birmingham; A. Redford, *Borough and City: The History of Local Government in Manchester: vol. II* (London, 1940) for Manchester and W.A. Robson, 'Drainage and Sewerage Services', *The Government and Misgovernment of London* (London, 1939) for London.

[16]   A.L. Dakyns, 'The Water Supply of English Towns in 1846', *Manchester School*, 2 (1931), 18–26; J.A. Hassan, 'The Growth and Impact of the British Water Industry in the Nineteenth century', *Economic History Review*, 38 (1985), 531–47.

[17]   A.S. Wohl, *Endangered Lives. Public Health in Victorian Britain* (London, 1983).

had the administrative resources to obtain powers to issue their own stock on the regional stock exchanges, larger towns probably did not face the same financial constraints as the smaller towns which were forced to resort to loans from the Public Works Loan Commissioners. The costs of such loans were high. Even when the 1875 Public Health Act and Public Loans Act provided blanket borrowing powers and unlimited access to the Loan Commissioners' funds, these carried a (then punitive) 5 per cent interest rate and a repayment period of twenty years which was much shorter than was reasonable for the long-lived assets under construction. It was not until the end of the nineteenth century that access to funds was eased by the activities of the new arm of central government, the Local Government Office.[18]

Measuring the impact of public health spending

How was the pattern of local government spending on public health and particularly its delay until the end of the nineteenth century, related to contemporary trends in mortality? The long-term trend of declining mortality under way in Britain from the eighteenth century stagnated during the phase of most intense industrialisation and urbanisation in the early nineteenth century. It was not until the 1870s that mortality once again began to decline amongst selected groups and it was very late in the century before the decline was universal across all age groups. Given this pattern it would appear that public health reforms could not have been responsible for the initial stages of nineteenth-century mortality decline. The period of peak investment in sanitary infrastructure occurred considerably after limited mortality decline had resumed in the 1870s. It is likely, however, that public health's contribution to mortality decline was significant in a regulatory sense well before the positive impact of a completed sanitary infrastructure at the end of the century. Environmental regulation was the daily work of a wide array of sanitary and medical personnel whose job it was to police the local environment in accordance with locally determined by-laws. From the 1840s an increasing battery of powers was being utilised by local councils, enabling them to plan and regulate the future development of their towns and to ensure standards of quality and healthfulness. The influence of the regulatory work overseen by local boards of health may well have been a significant component of early mortality decline. Clearly this effect will not be captured by our data on spending levels.

---

[18]   Wilson, 'The Finance of Municipal Capital Expenditure'.

Table 9.3: Changes in living standards, public health expenditures and mortality 1874–1913 (annual averages for 36 towns)*

	1874–77 (112 obs)*	1910–13 (100 obs)*	% Increase
Mortality per '000 (standardised)	22.1	17.0	-23.1
Population	87986	149650	70.0
Acreage	3704	6080	64.1
No. of inhabited houses	16107	31962	98.4
Price of land (rateable value per acre in £)	94.5	113.0	19.6
Weekly rent in pence for a 4-room house	64.4	59.8	-7.1
Food bundle (price in pence)	14.9	12.2	-18.3
Weekly wages of bricklayers in pence	430.3	476.4	10.7
Tax base (rateable value per head of population in £)	3.52	4.89	38.9
Local authority current expenditure in £ on:			
Water supply	19302	25286	31.0
Sewers	5575	12901	131.5
All sanitation	64214	133670	108.2
Local authority income from water rates in £ per head of population	0.205	0.369	80.0

* 36 towns for 4 years would yield 144 observations but data was missing for some towns which were therefore excluded.

Sources and definitions: The data relates to the area within the jurisdictional boundaries of the towns as municipal boroughs, that is, as administrative units of local government. The first four rows are extrapolated from Census of Population data. The standardised mortality rate for each town is given in the censuses and is estimated by applying the age distribution of the national population to the age-specific death rate for that town. The entries for rents, prices and wages are based on the Board of Trade report (1908) on the cost of living across towns in 1905, extrapolated back by the use of national indexes of average weekly wages, rents and prices.[19] The food bundle covers 4lb of bread, 7 lb. of potatoes and 3 eggs. All the rest of the data came from the Local Taxation Returns.

The scenes of squalor portrayed in Wohl's *Endangered Lives* appear to have been typical of most industrial towns at mid-century.[20] Numerous factors have been implicated as contributors to the stubbornly stationary and, in some places, increasing levels of mortality affecting urban centres. A variety of other factors have been lauded as the triggers and propellants of decline from the 1870s. Demographers have been able to show a close association between mortality levels and population density. Some of the best work here has been undertaken by Woods and Hinde, who examined life expectancy at birth in more than 600 registration districts in England and Wales in 1861.[21] It was found that there was a general tendency for life expectancy to be lower, the higher was the population density. A similar link was found between infant mortality and density. It is apparent from Table 9.1 that the high-density registration districts like Liverpool, Bristol and Leicester had much higher mortality levels in 1871 than those found in the benign rural townships of Richmond, Shaftesbury and Louth. But the relationship was clearly not a simple one. Carlisle, Preston, Swansea and Northampton registration districts all had relatively high mortality levels but relatively low density. Woods acknowledged such variations on the main theme and that there were other factors than density at work. Indeed, with Woodward he sketched out a model of likely causation in the introduction to their important edited volume *Urban Disease and Mortality*.[22] Socio-economic factors perceived as potentially important in this model included the standard of living, the wage-labour system, the sanitary infrastructure and the state of hospitals. Such complex interrelationships between these and other factors have not previously been subject to quantification and empirical analysis. Here, based on our sample of thirty-six towns in the period 1870–1914, we begin to undertake the task.

The trends in some key social and economic variables influencing mortality in the period 1870–1914 are shown in Table 9.3. The period under review is quite long, but was characterised by unambiguously rising living standards.

---

[19]   See Millward and Sheard, 'The Urban Fiscal Problem 1870–1914', pp. 529–32.
[20]   A. S. Wohl, *Endangered Lives*.
[21]   R. I. Woods and R. Hinde, 'Mortality in Victorian England: Models and Patterns', *Journal of Interdisciplinary History*, 18 (1987), 27–54, pp. 48–9.
[22]   Woods and Woodward, *Urban Disease and Mortality*.

Wages rose over the whole period, though from the early 1870s to the early 1890s they were actually constant when prices fell by about 30 per cent. The 1890s saw the first signs of wages and prices rising which they continued to do up to 1914. Population rose by about 30 per cent in both sub-periods but the housing stock rose noticeably more in the second period. Finally, whilst local authority expenditure on water supply per head of population rose by huge amounts initially and rather more gradually thereafter, the experience of sewers and other sanitation expenditure was quite the reverse, as we noticed earlier for capital expenditure. The question remains, how precisely were these changes in living standards, in the sanitary system and in population densities related to mortality decline in the period 1870–1914?

Our identification of underlying trends in key factors has helped to suggest whether their individual influence on mortality was likely to have been positive or negative but it has not determined the relative contribution of each factor to actual mortality decline. The strength with which different factors influenced mortality was by no means necessarily related to their rate of increase over time. Whilst the average number of inhabited houses in our towns expanded by 98 per cent between 1874/77 and 1910/13 it is possible that this increase was less significant in its impact on mortality than a proportionally much smaller rise in another factor. To calculate the strength with which different factors influenced mortality we have undertaken a statistical analysis of the association between mortality and the various factors affecting it. This multiple regression analysis enables the disaggregation of factors influencing mortality and measurement of the separate influence of each on mortality. It will not be discussed in detail, but some of the main findings will be described towards the end of the chapter.

The role of economic forces

Our measurement of the relative contribution of different factors to mortality decline recognises and distinguishes between two separate but complementary ways of viewing causation. The first recognises that mortality, as an outcome, was the product of a variable relationship between individuals and their physical environment. There is a biological process by which mortality follows from illness, which is itself a product of the balance between exposure and resistance to disease. We know that the virulence of disease changed little in the nineteenth century. Scarlet fever was the exception and had all but disappeared by the 1880s. Similarly, advances in medical practice had no noticeable impact on mortality, even in the case of simple improvements in obstetric aid whose potential importance for maternal mortality was enormous.[23] In effect the proximate 'causes' of mortality and its decline lay in three possible mechanisms. Improvements in nutrition may have raised resistance to infection, improvements in the sanitary infrastructure and in food quality controls may have reduced exposure to food and water-borne diseases and finally, the alleviation of living congestion by better town planning and better housing may have reduced exposure to airborne diseases like tuberculosis. Changes over time in the physical world facing individuals could alter both the extent to which they were exposed to infection and the degree to which they were susceptible to suffering fatally from disease. Mortality decline in the nineteenth century can be viewed as the result of beneficial changes in exposure and resistance, both of which reduced the severity with which physical factors depressed health. Spending by town councils and individuals on goods and services beneficial to health were potentially influential in improving life chances. Our regression analysis attempts to measure changes over time in different elements of the physical environment (particularly sanitary capacity) and to calculate the overall impact on actual mortality decline of local government investment in public health. The regression results are shown in Table 9.4.[24]

The first column of figures shows the 'impact effect' on mortality of each of the factors listed on the left-hand side. It shows how in general, across the full sample, an increase in for example the housing stock, affected mortality levels. Positive values indicate that an increase would have the effect of raising mortality whereas negative values indicate that an increase would reduce mortality. The second column of figures shows the actual percentage growth of the factors in question from the mid-1880s to the middle of the first decade of the new century. Multiplying the one by the other yields the third column, which essentially tells us the contribution of each factor to the overall fall in the crude death rate.

The results reveal that a rise of 10 per cent in the housing stock, with everything including population and town boundaries remaining unchanged, would generally have reduced mortality levels by some 4.58 per cent. In the

---

[23]   I. Loudon, 'Maternal Mortality: 1880–1950. Some Regional and International Comparisons', *Social History of Medicine*, 1 (1988), 183–223.

[24]   See Millward and Bell, 'Economic Factors in the Decline of Mortality' for a more detailed discussion of the regression analysis. The particular results reported in Tables 9.4 and 9.5 relate to the sample of towns over the twenty-eight years 1884–1911. In ten instances, however, the data was absent so the number of observations was 998 rather than the maximum of 36 x 28 = 1,008. A group effects model was used, with an adjustment for auto correlation. For details write to the authors. The sources for some of the data can be found in Table 9.3. The 1870s were excluded because the best proxy we had for sanitary and water supply capacities was data, in the Local Taxation Returns, on outstanding loans which are not available before the financial year 1883/84.

context of the mid- to late nineteenth century, town councils were increasingly utilising powers to regulate building. Local building by-laws began to contain requirements relating to space and ventilation and, increasingly, the design of houses began to take into account waste removal issues. It was not always at the legal insistence of an efficient town council that minimum building standards were imposed. In certain cases landowners themselves demonstrated a desire to improve the quality of local dwellings. In selling off a section of land to independent builders in Preston, William and Thomas Thomlinson wrote into all sales agreements that there were to be no back-to-back or back-and-front houses constructed; that all dwellings should exceed 15 feet in width; that they should have only two storeys and were to be designed for the accommodation of one family only.[25] The addition of new and better-quality housing to existing stocks may have increased average living space, reduced levels of exposure and have been better served by sanitary facilities.

The effect of population density on mortality was found to be captured best by town acreage related to the child population, measured as the number of five- to fifteen-year-olds.[26] An increase in children in the population was found to have a positive relationship with mortality. In this period a rise of 10 per cent in the number of five- to fifteen-year-olds with other factors unchanged would on average have led to a 2.35 per cent rise in mortality. In the period 1884/7 to 1906/9 an 18 per cent increase in the number of children took place which would have had the effect of raising mortality by 4.4 per cent had it not been for the concomitant influence of other factors tending to reduce mortality.

The contribution of alterations in food intake to changing mortality levels are extremely difficult to measure, given a general lack of recorded evidence on diet.[27] In our analysis we use as a proxy measure of diets in each town, the size of the food bundle which *could* be purchased with contemporary wage levels in each town. This is a far from ideal measure of the effect of nutritional change as McKeown has emphasised. As a factor, food does appear to have played a part in the decline of mortality though its impact was considerably weaker than that of housing. It is clear from Table 9.4 that improvements in sanitary infrastructure played only a modest role in mortality decline. As we have already stressed, concentrated investment in infrastructure occurred quite late in

---

[25]   N. Morgan, *An Introduction to The Social History of Housing in Victorian Preston* (Preston, 1983), p. 46.

[26]   The child data was interpolated from the Censuses of Population.

[27]   See D.J. Oddy, 'Food, Drink and Nutrition', in F.M.L. Thompson (ed.), *The Cambridge Social History of Britain 1750–1950: Vol. 2: People and their Environment* (Cambridge, 1990) for a discussion of the limitations of existing evidence.

Table 9.4: The contribution of changes in population densities, food and sanitation to the decline of mortality

Item	Impact effect on mortality	% change 1884/7 to 1906/9	Contribution to % change in mortality 1884/7 to 1906/9
No. children	0.235	18.5	4.3
Land area	0.118	4.2	0.5
No. houses	-0.458	44.4	-20.3
Food bundle	-0.194	18.5	-3.6
Sewer capacity	-0.004	97.5	-0.4
Street sanitary capacity	-0.004	220.0	-0.9
Other sanitary capacity	0.002	224.8	0.4
Water capacity	0.002	115.4	0.2
Sub-total			**-19.8**
Decade dummies			
1891–1900	0.006		0.6
1901–11	-0.057		-5.7
Total			**-24.9**
Actual death rate		-26.4	

the century and consequently it cannot explain mortality decline in the 1880s and early 1890s. The influence of improved sanitation is measured here by using sanitary expenditure as a proxy for sanitary capacity. This does not encompass the influence of regulation on mortality, which was an important element of public health programmes. As a result of this omission, which is unavoidable given the lack of a reliable proxy, our model probably underestimates the overall effect of public health spending on mortality levels. This said, some of the benefits of improvements in housing such as their size, quality and facility would have been contingent on developments both in sanitary infrastructure and building regulation. Housing may well be gaining some of the credit that is actually due to sanitation and public health.

Our regression includes two 'decadal dummies', which are designed to pick up the effects of special circumstances. In the 1890s infantile diarrhoea rose dramatically during several hot summers, whilst in the early years of the twentieth century infant mortality fell dramatically. Both incidents had a significant effect on the pattern of mortality in our sample, which is reflected in the values registered by them. Overall the factors included in our regression accounted for 94 per cent of the actual decline in mortality which took place in our sample of towns during the period 1884/87–1906/9. Whereas mortality actually declined by 26.4 per cent over the period, our model predicted a decline of 24.9 per cent.

A second and complementary approach to causation is to recognise that, whilst it was via their physical environment that the health of individuals (and thus mortality levels) were affected, factors such as the housing stock, food availability and the quality of sanitary facilities were not autonomous elements. They existed as the outcomes of decisions made by individuals and town councils, which involved often painful economic choices – the decision to spend on one thing rather than another. To view causation in this way is to acknowledge the importance of the influences that shaped decisions to spend on the physical environment and thereby affected the health of individuals.

Through the economic choices that they made, town councils and individuals had a capacity to alter aspects of the physical environment and, to an extent, their own position in relationship to it. Though most choices were influenced and informed by personal and cultural preferences, the outcome of the majority of decisions was determined by financial factors. The range of choices available was usually constrained by the financial resources available. By examining the relationship between mortality patterns in our sample towns and movements in incomes and prices our second regression model attempts to measure how strongly these factors influenced decisions to spend.

How households and town councils spent their money was influenced by the 'prices' they had to pay for health-enhancing goods and services. Households could improve their health environment by choosing to spend on a range of beneficial goods and services.[28] However, the higher the cost of good-quality foods, piped water, sewer rates, soap, and the installation water closets, the less inclined would households be to spend on these items. Less-congested dwelling areas would reduce the rate of exposure to disease but a family's ability to do anything about their accommodation would depend on the level of house rents and/or the price of land. Analogously, the decisions of town councils to construct sewers, waterworks and other sanitary facilities would be affected by the construction and running costs per mile of sewer and water mains and the

---

[28]   N. Tomes, 'The Private Side of Public Health: Sanitary Science, Domestic Hygiene and the Germ theory, 1870–1900', *Bulletin of the History of Medicine*, 64 (1990), 509–39.

costs per cubic capacity of reservoir water. In general, prices could be expected to have a *positive* relationship with mortality. Increasing prices for WCs, rent, soap and other goods would deter households from spending on them. Similarly, high costs per mile for sewer and water pipes would affect town council expenditure on these items. The effect of prices was especially relevant in the nineteenth century as rapidly diminishing returns characterised the expansion of water supplies and waste disposal systems. The resource costs of water and waste disposal are likely to have risen relative to other commodities and services because technological advances in water and waste disposal were not sufficient to counteract the effect of huge population increases on a constant resource base.

At present, apart from rents, we have only proxy measures of the resource costs of services. Data from the Local Taxation Returns on rateable values per acre provide an approximation of the price of land in each town. Town Council water receipts provide the basis for estimates of the price per gallon for water. By dividing receipts by the population we arrive at a figure for water income per head, variations in which provide some indication of how water prices changed. The measurement of sewer costs per mile is problematic given a lack of data on the mileage of mains. Data is available on the 'adopted' street mileage of each town, but not until after 1903. As an alternative, town council current expenditure on sewers and other sanitary facilities can be expressed per head of population. This provides a guide to variations existing across towns and over time in the sewer rates faced by households and in the costs per mile and per household for sewers and other sanitary facilities provided by town councils.

The other key element that influenced the outcome of decisions was the ability to spend, which was determined by income levels. An increase in income and thereby in the ability to spend would have the effect of *reducing* mortality, by enabling households to purchase a greater quantity of goods and services and by enabling councils to spend larger amounts on reform programmes. In our regressions we use data on bricklayers' weekly wages to measure household incomes.[29] How much a town council could spend on sewers depended on how much tax it could raise. Data from the Local Taxation Returns on rateable values per head provide our measure of the tax base in each town, the size of which one might expect to be *negatively* related to mortality. That is, other things being equal, a large tax base would be associated with lower mortality because it enabled higher spending on public health activities.

---

[29] Bricklaying was a wage-earning occupation found in most towns and regions and detailed data on the wages paid is available in our sources.

Table 9.5: The contribution of economic changes to the decline of mortality

Item	Impact Effect on mortality	% change 1884/7 to 1906/9	Contribution to % change in mortality 1884/7 to 1906/9
Tax base	-0.043	19.5	-0.8
Household income	-2.689	17.0	-45.7
Coal prices	0.378	35.8	13.5
Food prices	0.313	-1.6	-0.5
Rents	0.905	7.2	6.5
Sewer costs p.c.	0.005	116.4	0.6
Water costs p.c.	0.012	35.5	0.4
Sub-total			**-26.0**
Decade dummies			
1891–1900	0.017		1.7
1901–11	-0.032		-3.2
Total			**-27.5**
Actual death rate		-26.4	

The results of the second regression are shown in Table 9.5, which has the same structure as Table 9.4. Rents and coal prices both rose in the period 1884/87–1906/9, thereby significantly increasing the cost of access to living space and of keeping it warm. In contrast, the size of the tax base rose and food prices fell, both of which were forces making for a decline in mortality by encouraging individuals and councils to spend on beneficial goods and services. The most significant element was a rise in household incomes, which facilitated a rise in household expenditure on the complete range of health-enhancing goods. The prices of water and of sewers proved to have fairly weak effects, which may be reflecting difficulties in measuring the unit costs of these items, though it may also indicate that despite spiralling costs councils had little choice but to invest in essential facilities.

Our regression model slightly overpredicts the extent of mortality decline occurring in the period 1884/87–1906/9. Changing income and prices levels clearly appear to have influenced the spending patterns of individuals and town councils via the mechanisms outlined. What the model successfully provides is an impression of the economic context in which town councils made their decisions about important elements of public health expenditure. Equally successfully it charts movements in income and price forces which determined the abilities of individuals and households to purchase goods and services beneficial to their personal health chances.

Conclusion

The nineteenth century witnessed a huge expansion in the scale of local government expenditure generally. Our detailed examination of spending patterns has shown that by the end of the century public health had come to assume the largest single share of local authority expenditure which, at three-quarters of the total, placed expanded public health effort at the heart of the financial strains facing councils. The pace of investment in different services varied, though water was firmly established as the lead utility in terms of the timing and scale of investment. The period of peak investment in all services lay firmly at the end of the nineteenth century. The delay in expenditure until this late date was the outcome of a combination of practical, financial and technological difficulties, which had to be worked through and overcome by local councils.

When related to measures of population, density, housing, wages and prices, data from the Local Taxation Returns helps to describe the context in which local government officials made their decisions about public health issues and illuminates their responses to public health problems. However, the Local Taxation Returns data, which establishes the date at which expenditure on different services took place, does not indicate the point at which utilities became operational and began to have an impact on health. Ultimately, the late timing of peak investment established by our expenditure data discourages us from assigning significance to investment on infrastructure as a cause of mortality decline before the end of the nineteenth century. Our regression results confirm that increasing water, sewer and general sanitary capacities had only a weak influence on mortality before 1900.

The role of public health is not being fully and directly captured by our expenditure variables. Environmental regulation as an aspect of public health reform is not a factor which is formally measured by our model but it is a feature which is strongly emphasised by the strength of our housing variable. A 44.4 per cent increase in the existing housing stock was shown to be the factor in the physical environment most strongly influencing mortality patterns in the period 1884/87 to 1906/9. The significance of expansion in the housing stock was that new houses were increasingly subject to more stringent regulations in terms of space, ventilation and drainage, and had access to sewers and piped water. There were mandatory provisions with respect to new housing in the legislation as early as the 1840s and many towns supplemented these with their own by-laws.[30]

The measure of housing in our work is simply the number of occupied dwellings recorded in the census. Average occupancy fell over the period of investigation, but in our sample it was only by about 0.5 persons per house. It is likely that the improved *quality* of housing was probably the more important aspect of housing's beneficial effect on mortality. Much of the positive impact of housing was contingent on the presence of WCs and connections to sewers and piped water supplies. It appears that in our results housing is receiving credit that actually belongs to increased expenditure on public health infrastructure and tighter regulation of building quality.

The significant role of economic factors in the decline of mortality is made clear by our analysis of the relationships between income and price trends and patterns of mortality. Data shows that both household and council incomes increased considerably, which suggests that opportunities for investment improved. However, the unit costs of water and sewerage provision appear to have rocketed and any benefits from declining food prices were offset by increases in average rents and coal prices. Council spending on sanitary infrastructure appears to have been influenced more by the extent of increases in council tax bases than by the costs of sewers and the price of land, though this may be partly reflecting the limited data we have on 'price' effects, such as sewer costs per mile.

It is clear that our models need to be supplemented and improved by more data in order to capture fully the factors responsible for mortality decline and the mechanisms by which they operated. By the turn of the century a considerable sanitation capacity had been established and large expenditures on sewers, water and other sanitary capacity were to be found in many of the towns. It is difficult to avoid the provisional conclusion that this established sanitary capacity was a key element in allowing mortality to fall by large amounts in the 1890s and especially in facilitating the precipitous fall in infant mortality in the early 1900s. However, difficulties of measurement continue to

---

[30] Metropolis Building Act 1844, 7 and 8 Vict., c.82, *Collections of the Public General Acts*, (1815–1921); Town Improvement Clauses Act 1847, 10 and 11, Vict., c.34, *Collections of the Public General Acts* (1815–1921); Public Health Act 1848, 11 and 12, Vict., c.63, *Collections of the Public General Acts* (1815–1921).

mask the full influence of public health reforms on mortality. In addition to better measures of price effects, comprehensive quality measures are required to enable quantification of the influence of environmental regulation on health. The incorporation of data on the mortality associated with different diseases and specific age groups offers a further possibility of shedding more light on the many issues still unresolved.

10

Economics and infant mortality decline in German towns, 1889–1912: household behaviour and public intervention

John C. Brown

For most of the countries of Western and Central Europe, the key to the rapid decline in mortality towards the end of the nineteenth century was the decline in infant mortality. Although various conditions, including a series of hot and dry summers, may have masked the beginning of the decline, by the First World War it was apparent that it was well under way in both England and Germany. The decline in infant mortality was of key importance for sustaining the decline in general mortality that began in the last third of the nineteenth century. It was also critical for the shift in the relative healthfulness of cities. Germany, in particular, experienced unfavourable rates of infant mortality that placed it ahead of such poorer countries as Italy throughout the period prior to the First World War. Indeed, at the turn of the century, no other developed country of Western Europe experienced such high infant mortality as Germany. However, by the First World War, it has been established that infant mortality in middle- to large-sized German towns had fallen to such an extent that it was actually lower than in small towns and rural areas.[1] Figure 10.1 summarises the decline for about forty-five larger German cities with a population over 50,000 in the late 1880s. From an average of about 230 per 1,000 live births in the early 1890s, infant mortality remained relatively constant until the turn of the century, when it began a rather precipitous decline. By 1912, it had fallen almost 40 per cent.

---

[1]   See R.I. Woods, P.A. Watterson and J.H. Woodward, 'The Causes of Rapid Infant Mortality Decline in England and Wales, 1861–1921, Part I', *Population Studies*, 42 (1988), 343–66, p. 349 and J. Vögele, 'Urban Infant Mortality in Imperial Germany', *Social History of Medicine*, 7 (1994), 401–25.

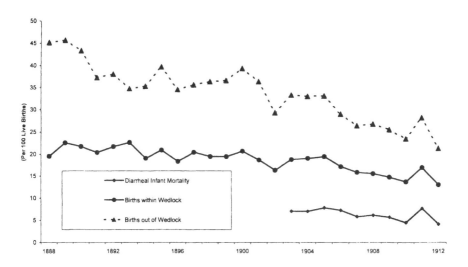

Figure 10.1: Infant mortality in German cities 1888–1912 (per 100 live births)

Source: *Statististisches Jahrbuch deutscher Städte, Preussische Statistik,* and *Medizinal-statistische Mitteilungen aus dem kaiserlichen Gesundheitsamt.*

Explaining the decline in infant mortality

Aside from offering a particular example of dramatic mortality decline, the case of Germany also highlights some of the key points at issue in explaining the decline in infant mortality throughout Europe and the United States during this period. The excellent surveys by Woods et al. and Vögele offer the salient explanations that have appeared in recent histories of public health and mortality.[2] The data from Great Britain (and to a lesser extent, Germany) suggests that a decline in neonatal mortality, which may have come about from an improvement in the health of the mother or higher birth-weights of infants, most likely does not play the leading role in the period before 1914. Instead, the efforts to explain the decline usually attempt to answer the standard questions that arise when attempting to understand the causes of morbidity and mortality in general: what were the sources of exposure to infection and what influences contributed to the ability of the infant to resist infection?

---

[2]   Woods et al., 'Causes', Part I; *idem* Part II, *Population Studies*, 42 (1989), 113–132; Vögele, 'Urban Infant Mortality'.

The answers to these questions typically stem from catalogues of possible causes compiled by contemporary observers and later historians.[3] The external environment (water supply and drainage) and the home environment (cleanliness) both may have contributed to the infant's exposure to disease. Aside from influencing cleanliness, parental care may have also influenced the infant's ability to resist infections through the direct route of breastfeeding, or through the indirect route of providing the appropriate responses to infant illness. Finally, changes in fertility or breastfeeding practices that led to longer birth intervals may have improved the prospects of the infant surviving because of better parental care.[4]

Two kinds of evidence are drawn upon to evaluate these proposed explanations, but there is still not any overall consensus. Most of the methodological innovation has been focused upon overcoming the limitations of the first approach, which simply looks at correlations taken at the same time across geographic units of observation or social classes. The problem with this approach to analysis is well known. The direct impact of certain influences, such as income, may explain much of the cross-sectional variation in infant mortality without being able to account for the rapid decline over time. Multiple regression implementations of this approach have identified candidate influences that may have been important at a particular point in time and that may have changed rapidly over the period of the initial decline, such as the level of education of women. Individual case-studies of cities (or countries) attempt to get around this problem by focusing on the timing of changes in one of the commonly-accepted potential explanations and then assessing whether it may or may not have occurred simultaneously or prior to the decline in infant mortality. These studies must also examine whether the change in the factor would have been sufficient to prompt the decline. In the case of Germany, only

---

[3]   See Woods et al., 'Causes' part 2, p. 114 for an example from the British doctor Newsholme.

[4]   See H. Kintner, 'The Determinants of Infant Mortality in Germany from 1871 to 1933' (unpublished PhD thesis, University of Michigan, 1982), *idem*, 'Determinants of Temporal and Areal Variations in Infant Mortality in Germany, 1871–1933', *Demography*, 25 (1988), 597–609. Although the point would seem obvious, the literature that has examined this question using both modern and historical data has arrived at mixed results. The case appears to be strongest for an important impact of birth interval length on the survival of neonates (M.A. Koenig, J.F. Phillips, O.M. Campbell and S. D'Souza, 'Birth Intervals and Child Mortality in Rural Bangladesh', *Demography*, 27 (1990), 251–65, p. 260), although some studies also find an important influence for birth intervals smaller than twelve months (A. Pebley, A. Hermalin and J. Knodel, 'Birth Spacing and Infant Mortality: Evidence for Eighteenth and Nineteenth Century German Villages', *Journal of Biosocial Science*, 23 (1991), 445–59 and S.L. Curtis, I. Diamond and J.W. McDonald, 'Birth Interval and Family Effects on Postneonatal Mortality in Brazil', *Demography*, 30 (1993), 33–43). K.A. Lynch and J.B. Greenhouse, 'Risk Factors for Infant Mortality in Nineteenth-Century Sweden', *Population Studies*, 48 (1994), 117–33, find that the length of birth intervals had virtually no influence on infant mortality in historical Swedish data.

one study has applied multiple regression analysis to cross-section time series data in an effort to uncover the role of important influences behind the decline in infant mortality over the period 1871 to 1933. Although the variables used 'explained' over three-quarters of the sample variance, the ability to predict the actual decline in infant mortality was limited to the rate of marital fertility and the per capita coverage of infant welfare centres. Kintner's estimates imply that the decline in marital fertility from 1871 to 1933 would account for about four-fifths of the decline, and the widened coverage of infant welfare centres would account for another one-fifth.[5] Unfortunately, for reasons to be noted momentarily, the results say perhaps more about the difficulty of addressing the decline of infant mortality with multiple regression techniques than they do about the actual causes behind the decline.

The final approach can include both the cross-sectional and the time series data used in the two prior approaches. It increases the burden of evidence needed to test an explanation by taking a closer look at the causes of infant death.[6] Although in the case of England, mortality from gastrointestinal disease appears to be more of a nuisance in identifying the 'true' sources of decline than something to be explained in its own right, in Germany (and, apparently, also the United States) it was a key contribution to infant mortality. The German data suggests the share was in the order of one-third to one-half for Germany and Prussia, and about 37 percent for large German cities before the First World War.[7] Vögele's work offers a critique of the notion, for example, that improvements in the sanitary quality of urban milk supplies mattered for the decline in infant mortality before 1914, by noting that the introduction of

---

[5]   Arguing that short-term changes in summer temperature and precipitation spuriously inflated the mortality from diarrhoeal disease, Woods et al., 'Causes', direct most of their attention to the decline in non-diarrhoeal disease. S. Szreter, 'The Importance of Social Intervention in Britain's Mortality Decline c. 1850–1914: A Re-interpretation of the Role of Public Health', *Social History of Medicine*, 1 (1988), 1–37 argues that the share of diarrhoeal disease of about 20 per cent in urban counties appearing in the cause of death statistics is too low and should include a share of deaths due to convulsions. S. Guha, 'The Importance of Social Intervention in England's Mortality Decline: The Evidence Reviewed', *Social History of Medicine*, 7 (1994), 89–113, pp. 107–11 argues that the classification schemes remained so unstable during the late nineteenth century that any time series evidence based upon the official cause of death statistics is bound to be subject to wide margins of error. The debate in Germany over the appropriate assignment of *Krämpfe* (cramps) has similar tones, particularly when Prussian cause of death statistics are being used. See Kintner, 'Determinants', pp. 602ff. These conclusions are based on Kintner's presentation of her regression results and the data in Table 10.2.

[6]   See Kintner, 'Determinants of Infant Mortality' and Vögele, 'Urban Infant Mortality'.

[7]   See R. Spree, 'On Infant Mortality Change in Germany since the Early 19th Century', Mimeo (Munich, 1995), p. 12, Kintner, 'Determinants of Infant Mortality', p. 157 and Vögele, 'Urban Infant Mortality', p. 408. A regression of the mean annual infant mortality on the infant mortality from diarrhoeal diseases in ninety-four towns explains about two-thirds of the variance: Infant Mortality=121.7+1.21*Diarrhoeal Mortality. The t-statistic is 33.2 on Diarrhoeal Mortality.

improved milk supplies prompted few reductions in tuberculosis mortality or the well-known peak in summer infant mortality.

Economic behaviour and infant mortality decline

Although the basic model of exposure and resistance serves well to highlight some of the key epidemiological issues at stake in understanding infant mortality decline, it may be less well suited to understanding the contribution of the social and economic influences that feature prominently in many discussions. A case in point is Kintner's finding of the overwhelming influence of marital fertility in explaining infant mortality in Germany. Her statistical approach (and efforts to look solely at the correlation of infant mortality and fertility) would imply that the gains from increasing birth intervals alone in the wake of fertility decline (and perhaps the proportional increase in resources available for the remaining children) could cause massive reductions in infant deaths: a conclusion that can not be sustained by the statistical work carried out on detailed, individual-level data as cited at length in note 4. The problem is that a large part of the correlation between infant mortality and fertility may well be spurious, if other (unmeasured) influences acted both upon marital fertility and infant mortality.[8] An increase in the value of women's time or in the couple's valuation of the mother's health could, for example, prompt an attempt to reduce the number of pregnancies. If a family's intentions with respect to final family size remained unchanged, it would also be expected that the household (or woman) would seek out better ways of caring for the children who had already been born. Although the proximate cause would appear to be biological, the actual source of the decline in infant mortality would be found in changes in social or economic conditions. The solution to this problem is to more carefully model the causal relationships in order to identify those influences that are most likely to be truly external. Woods and his collaborators offer an example of taking greater care in modelling the potential links between fertility and infant mortality. Closer attention to modelling the household behaviour that may have contributed to infant mortality decline also helps to highlight the key debates in the historical literature over the sources of the decline in infant mortality.[9]

The economic models of household behaviour first pioneered by the economist Gary Becker and subsequently applied in a number of studies of household behaviour with respect to health and mortality offer a coherent

---

[8]   The term used to describe this kind of statistical problem is 'simultaneity bias'. Typically, the presence of simultaneity bias will lead to an exaggeration of the importance of the variable in question.

[9]   Woods et al., 'Causes of Rapid Infant Mortality Decline'.

approach to identifying other potential sources of such simultaneity bias.[10] Such a model posits household preferences over a number of 'goods' that it consumes, including the services of children. The preferences can be represented as a household utility function over the number of surviving children (C), or F (marital fertility) – M (infant and child mortality), other goods and food (X), and the leisure of the husband and wife, which is simply the total number of hours available to them (L) net of their work time, l_m or l_f :

(1) $U(X, F - M, L - l_m, L - l_f)$

Although the discussion here focuses on legitimate births, it can also include illegitimate births.

As would be obviously the case for the vast majority of families who experienced declining infant mortality, the family faces a number of constraints on its ability to meet the desired number of children who survive to maturity. The most important factor at the end of the nineteenth century is its ability to convert its purchase of market goods (and investment of its own time, if need be) into a home environment that will ensure that the infant survives and flourishes. One simple way of expressing this relationship is to note that the number of surviving children will depend upon the amount of time spent caring for them. Suppose that we summarise this time as B, or the amount of time spent breastfeeding the infant, although it can include time spent on other childcare as well. This time represents another claim on the leisure time remaining to the wife after working. In addition, the family may purchase goods on the market (pasteurised milk, for example) that could enhance the well-being of the infant. We can label these goods 'Z' goods. Finally, the family's choice of housing may also matter. One feature of housing that crops up repeatedly in the literature is the sanitary condition of the home, or S. It is also useful to incorporate factors beyond the household's control (ε), such as the temperature during the summertime, that may influence the ability of the family to meet its goal of a particular family size. If the technology that transforms these goods is g ($\cdot$), then

(2) $M = g(Z, S, B, \varepsilon)$

---

[10]   See the recent contribution by J. Mokyr and R. Stein, 'Science, Health, and Household Technology: The Effect of the Pasteur Revolution on Consumer Demand', in T. Bresnahan and R. Gordon (eds), *The Economics of New Goods* (Chicago, 1997). This discussion draws heavily upon their general formulation of the problem of mortality decline, although it differs from their strong emphasis on the germ theory of disease.

Finally, the family faces a budget constraint that reflects on the one side the costs of achieving what it desires in life and on the other, the resources available to it to meet those goals.

$$(3) \quad p_s S + X + p_z Z = w_m l_m + w_f (l_f - B)$$

The ps are simply the prices of the various goods. The price of X is set to one to ease interpretation of the other prices. The terms, w_m and w_f, are the potential wages earned by the husband and wife, respectively. Note that the more time the wife spends breastfeeding her child, the less time she has available for other work. Under the assumption of utility maximisation, the household ends up choosing the number of children, the goods X, Z and S, and the amount of time spent breastfeeding the infant and working in the labour market. The 'solution' to the household's decision-making points to some of the interrelationships that make the analysis of a complicated outcome, such as the survival of a child, particularly difficult.

Note first of all, that C^* (the number of surviving children) will in the final analysis depend only upon all of the factors outside of the household's control, including the wage earned by the husband and wife, the prices for sanitation and pasteurised milk, and the external environment. The same may be said of the other important decision variables of the household, including how long the mother would breastfeed and what kind of environment the child would be raised in. Second, treating the various decision variables that crop up in the literature as beyond the family's control, when they are in fact under the family's control, can lead to important biases in the evaluation of their influence on the decline in infant mortality.

Before reviewing some of the main conclusions of the literature on the decline in infant mortality, it is important to confront a common objection to the idea that families may have exerted any rational choice that influenced levels of fertility or mortality. One perspective may argue that working-class families at the turn of the century faced such desperate economic circumstances that they were beyond rational choice and were simply compelled by their poverty to accept the lot dealt them by fate. In reality, this kind of objection is well within the spirit of this simple model of household choice. The American Children's Bureau Surveys, which investigated the causes of infant mortality, found a striking inverse correlation between the earnings of the husband and the decision of the wife to work in the formal labour market. Once earnings of the husband were high enough, the family would almost invariably choose to have the wife remain in the home.[11] Choosing to work in the home rather than

---

[11]   See A. Rochester, *Infant Mortality. Results of a Field Study in Baltimore, Maryland* (Washington, DC, 1919), table 92 for data from a Baltimore study of the mortality experience of the entire population of infants born in a particular year. The share of mothers working

outside of the home displayed a similar pattern. As long as information is also available about infant mortality or fertility among families facing less financially-constrained circumstances, it is possible to incorporate the role of income in the analysis of infant mortality.

The other potential objection is more fundamental: the motivations of couples in nineteenth-century Europe may have differed fundamentally from the motivations of couples today. One line of reasoning that draws on this perspective is perfectly acceptable within the terms of the model of household behaviour. Many historians of the fertility decline that commenced in most of Europe during the final decades of the nineteenth century have argued that for most of historical time, reproductive decisions lay outside of the control of individual couples. Knodel and Van de Walle suggest, for example, that in the absence of birth control, infant mortality may have served as an exceptionally inefficient, yet ultimately successful form of family limitation.[12] The implication for the model would be that the couple felt that its control over M would need to be responsive to the number of children. In the formulation of the g ($\cdot$) function, another factor beyond the family's control would be the number of children (F). Infant mortality that resulted from neglect, or commonly-used but lethal feeding practices, could have also resulted from choice if the number of children was already too high.

Several authors stress another cause of infant mortality at the turn of the century: the ignorance and fecklessness of mothers.[13] Although mothers may have wished to 'secure the welfare of their offspring', as Newsholme so succinctly puts it, their ignorance about the appropriate approach to infant care, including their lack of understanding of the germ theory of disease, made it difficult for them to make informed decisions. As Mokyr and Stein express it, the g ($\cdot$) function for producing improved infant health was poorly understood. Imhof suggests a second kind of critique that would also undermine the

---

outside of the home during pregnancy declined dramatically with income. B.S. Duncan and E. Duke, *Infant Mortality. Results of a Field Study in Manchester, New Hampshire Based on Births in One Year* (Washington, DC, 1917), table 28 present similar results for the New England textile city of Manchester, New Hampshire and E. Hunter, *Infant Mortality. Results of a Field Study in Waterbury, Connecticut Based on Births in One Year* (Washington, D.C., 1917), Table 29 offers similar data for the Connecticut brass manufacturing centre of Waterbury.

[12]   J. Knodel and E. van de Walle, 'Lessons from the Past: Policy Implications of Historical Fertility Studies', in A.J. Coale and S. Cotts Watkins (eds), *The Decline of Fertility in Europe* (Princeton, 1986).

[13]   Mokyr and Stein, 'Science, Health, and Household Technology'; A. Newsholme, *Report by the Medical Officer on Infant and Child Mortality* (London, 1910), pp. 70–74; Woods et al., 'Causes of Rapid Infant Mortality Decline'; D.C. Ewbank and S. Preston, 'Personal Health Behaviour and the Decline in Infant and Child Mortality: The United States, 1900–1930', in J. Caldwell et al., *What do we know about the health transition?* (Canberra, Australia, 1990), pp. 116–49.

usefulness of this approach. Instead of individual decision-making conditioned by social mores, two fundamentally different attitudes towards life and death explain the differences in the regional pattern of infant mortality in Germany.[14] Areas that had been subject to the ravages of repeated wars, including the Thirty Years' War, adopted a fundamentally passive attitude towards life and infant death. The 'system of wastage' included a high-fertility, high-mortality regime that was found in southern and eastern Germany. The regions that had escaped most of the ravages of war adopted a fundamentally different perspective: the 'system of conservation of human life'. Neither of these systems represented 'rational choices', and they continued to inform infant care practices into the twentieth century. Vögele, while skeptical of Imhof's methodology, concurs that there needed to be a fundamental change in attitudes before infant mortality could decline. This was in turn prompted by an 'increase in the rationalist conduct of human life'.[15]

Interpreting competing explanations for the decline

The model captured by equations 1 to 3 offers a helpful framework for interpreting the leading explanations of the decline in infant mortality. It also points to some of the statistical problems inherent in attempting to establish causal links. Three potential sources of influence come to mind: the changes in economic structure and the increase in incomes associated with industrialisation, the actions of public authorities in the provision of health-enhancing goods at lower costs, and the efforts of public and private authorities to change the preferences of households (the utility function in 1) or the households' perceptions of the consequences of their behaviour on the health of their infants (the g $(\cdot)$ function in 2).

In terms of the model of household behaviour, industrialisation and urbanisation would be expected to influence the wages earned by both mother and father (w_f and w_m) as well as the prices paid for goods such as soap for the household (a Z-good) or food (an X-good). Although changes in the prices of these goods have received some attention, the chief focus has been the influence of changes in the wages paid to adult men and women. Consider, first, the impact of changes in earnings on the hours worked (l_f and l_m) and the hours spent breastfeeding (B). For married women, the argument can cut two ways. Based upon changes in the seasonality in infant deaths, Huck argues that industrialisation in northern England prompted rising earnings opportunities for women outside the home and led to higher rates of labour-force participation

---

[14]   A.M. Imhof, 'Unterschiedliche Säuglingssterblichkeit in Deutschland, 18. ... bis 20. Jahrhundert-Warum?' *Zeitschrift für Bevölkerungswissenschaft*, 7 (1981), 343–82.
[15]   Vögele, 'Urban Infant Mortality in Germany', p. 424.

for married women and reductions in breastfeeding, as the cost of an hour away from the workplace rose proportionately.[16] Kintner found that her estimate of the average duration of breastfeeding was inversely correlated with the female labour-force participation rate in non-agricultural occupations. Vögele notes that the increased resources received by the household from higher female earnings may have offset the impact of a lower value of B (or breastfeeding) with enhanced purchases of other goods, including the health-enhancing Z-goods such as soap or perhaps improved household sanitation. To the extent that illegitimacy also responded to enhanced earnings opportunities for women, higher wages for single women may have also influenced their willingness to have children without marriage, while at the same time exposing their offspring as illegitimate children, to much higher risks of mortality than if they were born within wedlock.[17]

The analysis of increased earnings of men is much more straightforward, since it does not imply tradeoffs for the household that would influence the survival of children. An increase in the wage would be expected to decrease the hours worked by women (l_f). In addition, it would increase the purchases of all goods, including the Z-goods and improved housing with better sanitation and more space. How much of the additional earnings would be allocated to such goods, and how much would be spent on tobacco or at the pub, would depend upon how the household valued children over other consumption. The contemporary literature in Germany is rife with suggestions about the preference orderings of working-class households, but it is not clear how accurate they actually are.

Since diarrhoeal diseases are transmitted primarily through physical contact with the excrement of a patient and only secondarily through polluted water supplies, it would appear that there would be some scope for improvements in access to better sanitation to have an impact on infant mortality. Before examining the 'household economics' of sanitary choice, it is important to see whether a case can be made at all for a role for sanitary improvement in infant

---

[16]   See P. Huck, 'Shifts in the Seasonality of Infant Deaths in Nine English Towns During the Ninteenth Century: A Case for Reduced Breastfeeding?', *Explorations in Economic History*, 34 (1997), 368–86. The contemporary and historical literature on the links between economic incentives and breastfeeding (and then child survival) is vast, if also plagued with simultaneity biases. See Woods et al., 'Causes of Rapid Infant Mortality Decline' for a discussion of some of the rather sparse evidence from England. H. Kintner, 'Trends and Regional Differences in Breastfeeding in Germany from 1871 to 1937', *Journal of Family History*, 10 (1985), 163–82 provides a nice summary of the data on breastfeeding that she culled from the surveys carried out at the time in Germany.

[17]   See Kintner, 'Trends and Regional Differences', p. 170 and Vögele, 'Urban Infant Mortality'. This discussion has not discussed the potential impact of changes in women's wages on fertility behaviour. It is possible that a higher valuation of women's time (for example, on the small farm) may have prompted extended breastfeeding as an approach to reducing the risk of pregnancy. See Knodel and van de Walle, 'Lessons'.

mortality decline. Two objections have been raised over the purported link between improvements of household consumption of sanitary conveniences and infant mortality decline: sanitary improvements of the late nineteenth century may not have been effective, and even if they were effective, the expansion of improvements does not coincide with the decline in infant mortality.

Most of the important historical debate over the sources of infant mortality decline has accepted the claims of physicians such as Newsholme that use of privies or pail closets could prompt higher infant mortality.[18] However, historians point to evidence that the time series of infant mortality in both England and Germany does not appear to coincide with the period of the great sanitary reforms undertaken during the last third of the nineteenth century.[19] Guha argues on the basis of evidence from two studies that diarrhoea was endemic to cities of the late nineteenth century and thus 'not controllable through Victorian sanitary measures'. Most infants would be subject to exposure from it and sanitary reform would offer little hope of removing the sources of that exposure since, primarily, the faecal–oral route spread the disease. A study from 1908 found that a comparison of two districts with widely differing sanitary conditions (privy and pail middens in one, water closets in the other) revealed little difference in the incidence of diarrhoea.[20] Although it is impossible to replicate the study cited by Guha, simple regression analysis of data on sanitary provision and mortality from diarrhoea and enteric fever found in Fletcher suggests that the issue is still open. As Table 10.1 suggests, the use of privy middens had a strong positive impact on mortality and morbidity, while the use of water closets generally reduced mortality. The small sample sizes for these regressions may diminish the strength of the predictions, but they still point in the direction suggested by Newsholme and other observers at the turn of the century.[21]

In addition to continued widespread use of privies, households in early twentieth-century Germany frequently shared the same toilet facilities, which increased the risk of the spread of diarrhoeal disease from the wider exposure of the family to sources outside the household. Table 10.2 summarises some of the data that could be gleaned from housing censuses and illustrates the extent of the problem. The high density of housing in western, southern, and eastern

---

[18]   Newsholme, *Infant and Child Mortality*, pp. 63–8.

[19]   See Vögele, 'Urban Infant Mortality'; Guha, 'Importance', pp. 111–12, and Szreter, 'Importance', pp. 28–9.

[20]   Guha, 'Importance of Social Intervention', pp. 110–12.

[21]   W.W.E. Fletcher, 'Report to the Local Government Board Upon the Sanitary Circumstances and Sanitary Administration of the City Borough of Middleborough' in *Reports to the Local Government Board on Public Health and Medical Subjects* (London, 1910), pp. 21–31.

Table 10.1: Influences of sanitary conditions on enteric fever and diarrhoea

Influence	Morbidity of enteric fever	Mortality from diarrhoea	Mortality from enteric fever
Share of privies	0.016	0.010	0.006
	(4.09)	(1.22)	(3.99)
Share of water closets	-0.031	-0.034	0.005
	(3.59)	(1.89)	(1.32)
Constant	0.777	1.19	0.073
	(6.68)	(6.30)	(2.73)
R^2	.50	.21	.77
N	16	16	9

Source: Results of ordinary least squares regressions corrected for heteroskedasticity. The data is from W.W.E. Fletcher, 'Report to the Local Government Board Upon the Sanitary Circumstances and Sanitary Administration of the City Borough of Middleborough' in *Reports to the Local Government Board on Public Health and Medical Subjects* (London, 1910), pp. 29–31.
Notes: *t*-statistics in parentheses.

Germany ensured that most families would live in an apartment block. Most building codes in effect before the First World War only required that one toilet be built for every two households. Since housing inspection programs were for the most part only becoming effective shortly before the First World War, large numbers of families continued to share facilities as a means of reducing the rent. At the turn of the century, from one-third to two-thirds of the households in these towns relied upon privies. Of course, the problem could be compounded in cities such as Augsburg, where until relatively late most families still relied upon privies and where a large share of households shared sanitary facilities with two or more other households. Although most apartment buildings were supplied with piped water by this time, the tap available could still be inconveniently located.

Certainly, for German cities, large numbers of families were served by the kinds of sanitary facilities that would increase the risk of transmission of disease by the faecal–oral route. Inconveniently located water supplies, privies, and large numbers of households sharing sanitary facilities would all increase the risk of infant diarrhoea. The classic definition of sanitary reform includes the provision of piped clean water to households and the removal of household

Table 10.2: Sanitary conditions of housing in urban Germany c. 1900

Sanitary feature	Munich 1904–7	Augsburg 1904	Düsseldorf 1905	Nuremburg 1901–2
Water supply in courtyard only	4	37	NA	20
Sewer connection	90	85	NA	90
Privy	20	98	79	98
One household per toilet	52	41	44	67
Three or more households per toilet	8	40	25	14

Source: H. Rost, *Die Wohnungsuntersuchung in der Stadt Augsburg vom 4.01. bis 24.03.04* (Augsburg, 1906); K. Buechel, *Ergebnisse der allgemeinen Wohunungsuntersuchung in Nürnberg 1901/02* (Nuremburg, 1907); Munich housing census sample and 'Die Grundstücks- und Wohnungszählung', *Mitteilungen zur Statistik der Stadt Düsseldorf*, 2 (1907).
Notes: The numbers refer to the share of households living in an apartment with the stated sanitary feature.

and human waste with a sewer system. In Germany and England it had two potential kinds of impact: a price effect and an enforced consumption effect. For most households, sanitary reform exploited economies of scale to lower the price of good-quality water, and perhaps as well, effective waste disposal. The reduced price for sanitary goods would be expected to have the usual effect on household usage of any good. In combination with rising incomes, it would be expected to increase the installation of water mains (and taps) in homes and increase the use of flush toilets. Sanitary reform also frequently required households to accept the water and sewer hook-ups, whether they wanted them or not. The enactment of building codes and housing use codes may have also increased the mandatory consumption of the newer sanitary facilities after the turn of the century. If these codes were binding, households would be consuming more (or better, and higher-priced) sanitary services than they would if they were able freely to choose their own housing mix. In Britain, the reports presented to the Local Government Board suggest that in practice there was still a considerable scope in many cities for families to choose a wide range of sanitary conditions, particularly with respect to sewage and toilet facilities. The housing censuses carried out by German cities suggest considerable variation as well. It should also be noted that government intervention may have actually slowed down the introduction of improved sanitation. Even at the turn of the century, concerns about water pollution prompted German cities to prohibit the introduction of human waste into sewage systems. As late as 1900, one-half of German cities continued to rely exclusively on privies for the disposal of human waste.

The evidence from the forty-seven largest German cities over the period 1888–1912 suggests that sanitary reform still had some room for improvement. Figure 10.2 presents the progress of sanitary reform according to three variables for these cities: the share of buildings equipped with piped water, the share of population connected to a sewer where water closets were also allowed, and the share of buildings receiving water supplies of improved quality (ground or spring water or water from an impoundment). The most dramatic progress occurred after 1900, as more cities invested in costly sewerage farms to provide for the disposal of raw sewage.

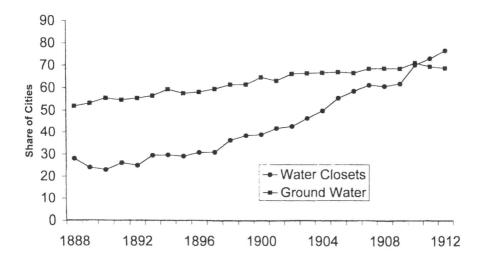

Figure 10.2: The progress of sanitary reform in German cities, 1888–1912

Source: *Statistisches Jahrbuch deutscher Städte*, E. Grahn, *Die städtische Wasserversorgung im Deutschen Reiche sowie in einigen Nachbarländern* (Munich and Berlin, 1898 and 1902) and H. Salomon, *Die städtische Abwasserbeseitigung in Deutschland*, vols 1–3 (Jena, 1906).
Notes: The share with ground water is the share of lots in the city. The share with water closets is the share of the population served by the sewer system with the right to use a water closet.

Household choices about infant care

While the historical literature has downplayed the potential role of improvements in sanitary conditions, it has increasingly emphasised the potential for important changes in household behaviour that may have substantially improved the survival probabilities of infants.[22] During the decade or so before the First World War, the infant health movement swept both Great Britain and the Continent. An important outgrowth of this movement was the efforts carried out by both private groups and governments to influence the care received by infants. The efforts took on many forms, but were concentrated on increasing breastfeeding, improving the quality and cleanliness of the food consumed by the infant after weaning, and providing instruction on the care of infants. The comments of Newsholme suggest an emphasis on hygiene at home. The German movement dispensed a wide range of advice in an effort to disabuse mothers of such practices as excessive swaddling of the infant or the depriving it of adequate fresh air. These efforts aimed at changing behaviour, both directly by reducing the cost to the family of providing good-quality care to the infant, and indirectly by attempting to influence the family's understanding of the consequences of its infant care practices.

In Germany, the primary focus after the turn of the century was on increasing the amount and length of breastfeeding. Under 10 per cent of mothers in the north and over one-half of mothers in the south never breastfed their infants. Municipalities typically undertook direct measures to encourage breastfeeding and offset the harmful effects of early weaning.[23] They included providing low-cost pasteurised milk at city milk dispensaries in an effort to lower the cost of a good-quality Z-good, milk, so that a mother would be better able to feed a weaned infant clean milk. In addition, a growing number of cities provided mothers with 'breastfeeding premia' to continue breastfeeding. The premia were designed to offset the potential cost (w_f*B) to the mother of devoting time to breastfeeding, although in reality the replacement was minimal. In the Bavarian industrial city of Fürth, a woman receiving the premia would be paid 5 marks after two months of continued breastfeeding and up to fifteen marks after four months. Receipt of the premia would be contingent on an examination at the local Mothers' Advice Centre. The wage paid to a female

---

[22]   See Ewbank and Preston, 'Personal Health'; Vögele, 'Urban Infant Mortality'; Woods et al., 'Causes', B. Thompson, 'Infant Mortality in Nineteenth-Century Bradford'; in R. Woods and J. Woodward (eds), *Urban Disease and Mortality in Nineteenth-Century England* (London, 1994); and Kintner, 'Determinants of Infant Mortality'.

[23]   See Kintner, 'Trends and Regional Differences' and G. Tugendreich, 'Öffentliches Kinderschutz', Th. Weyl (ed.), *Handbuch der Hygiene* (Leipzig, 1910) for more extended discussions of the infant welfare movement in Germany.

day labourer was 1.9 Marks in 1910. The premia thus would amount to less than 10 per cent of the potential earnings during the entire period.[24]

Aside from the narrower focus on provision of lower-cost milk and breastfeeding premia, the efforts in Germany aimed at changing mothers' minds about the most effective methods of infant care. This approach was an effort primarily aimed at educating parents about the appropriate shape of the g (·) function and, perhaps, changing parental attitudes towards their children (the utility function in 1). These efforts began with the mailing of a brochure on the proper care of the infant at birth and continued with visiting nurses, lectures and 'museums'. The provision of the premia was typically viewed as a way to coax the mothers inside the doors of the advice centres, where they would be provided with the full range of information on infant health care and encouraged to have their infant examined by a physician. In the best of cases, those visiting the advice centres or the infant welfare centres could constitute an appreciable number of the mothers in any one year. For example, by 1909 the seven Berlin centres had seen about one-third of the children born during that year, although the share seen while they were less than one month old was about one-sixth. In Fürth, the share of newborns visiting the centre was also about one-sixth.[25]

Figure 10.3 provides a fragmentary sketch of the rapid expansion of the infant welfare movement in the years shortly before 1914. Although there were only a few pioneers prior to 1900, by 1910 most of the larger cities in Germany for whom information is available had some form of infant welfare centres and/or milk dispensaries. The data in Figure 10.3 does not indicate the extent of the services within towns, but it does give some insight into the rapid expansion of the infant health movement and the coincidence of that expansion with the decline in infant mortality documented in Figure 10.1.

Placing the explanations for infant mortality decline in the historical literature in the context of the household decision-making model suggests three important methodological points about efforts to examine hypotheses. First, even if the simple household model is only a rough approximation of the potential causal mechanisms at work, sorting out the influence of various mechanisms on infant mortality poses a significant challenge and argues for as much care as possible in measuring the relevant variables. Consider the influence of an increase in the wage paid to women workers. The direct effect may be felt both in reduced breastfeeding, but also in increased household demand for an improved local environment. Analysis that includes the wages of women must of necessity note that some of its influence may be channelled

[24] See Haupstaatsarchiv Nürnberg, Regierung, K.d.I Abg. 168 Tit. V. Nr. 21 for the data on the premia offered in Fürth.
[25] See Tugendreich, 'Öffentliches Kinderschütz', p. 633 and Haupstaatsarchiv Nürnberg, Regierung, K.d.I Abg. 168 Tit. V. Nr. 21.

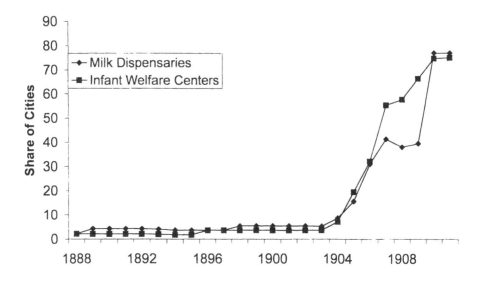

*Figure 10.3: The diffusion of infant welfare initiatives in German cities,
1888–1908*

Sources: *Statistisches Jahrbuch deutscher Städte*; G. Tugendreich, 'Öffentliches Kinderschutz',
Th. Weyl (ed.), *Handbuch der Hygiene* (Leipzig, 1910); A. Keller, 'Der Umfang der
Unterstützungen an stillenden Mütter', *Zeitschrift für Säuglingsschutz*, 1 (1909), 180–85, *idem*,
'Sozial-hygienische Einrichtungen: Deutschland', A. Keller and C. Klunker (eds), *Säuglingsf
ürsorge und Kinderschutz in den europäischen Staaten, Part 1* (Berlin, 1912) and 'Berichten
auf den Runderlass'.
Notes: The share of cities is the share of cities with one or more milk dispensaries or Infant
Welfare Centres.

through household purchases of improved sanitary conditions. An estimate of
the impact of increases in women's earnings would require inclusion of both
the direct and the indirect effect. Second, the model suggests that the data
should be examined for potential simultaneity bias. Finally, although the ideal
individual-level data for examining the problem of infant mortality decline may
not be available, the model does suggest working with as much disaggregated
data as possible. Given the dramatically different economic motivation for
children in the city as opposed to the rural areas, it would also seem sensible to
disaggregate the data by location. This analysis focuses on urban areas. In
addition, the motivation for and ability to provide infant care would be
expected to differ substantially between single mothers and married mothers.
Separating data on infant mortality into legitimate and illegitimate mortality
would thus seem appropriate. Finally, particularly in the case of Germany, the

determinants of diarrhoeal disease seem particularly important for influencing the course of infant mortality overall. Separate analysis of diarrhoeal disease should provide some ability to assess what was influencing infant mortality decline.

Statistical analysis of infant mortality in German towns

Fortunately, the efforts of local German statistical offices and the extensive contemporary research have permitted the collection of a data set that permits an empirical assessment of what may have accounted for infant mortality in urbanised Germany. The data set includes legitimate and illegitimate infant mortality for all German towns with a population greater than 50,000 over the period 1889 to 1912, when the decline in infant mortality took root in German cities (see Figure 10.1). In addition, it includes infant mortality due to diarrhoeal disease and other causes for all towns with a population greater than 50,000 from 1905 to 1912, and many of the large towns for 1903 and 1904.[26] The specification of the mortality relationship drew upon the various suggestions found in the empirical literature. In particular, it focused initially on variables that proxy for the economic influences suggested by the simple model of household choice: employment opportunities for women (measured by the presence of textile employment and the domination of heavy industry, which typically was inversely correlated with female employment) and the wage paid to female workers. The share of illegitimate births was also included; more illegitimate children would mean that they were not only to be found in the poorest (single mother) households. In addition, (exogenous) influences on infant mortality were also included: the average temperature during the months of June, July and August, and the rate of stillbirths per 1,000 births.[27] The share of mothers never breastfeeding was included to test for that influence on infant mortality.[28] Variables designed to capture the influence of

---

[26]   The mortality data come primarily from the *Statistisches Jahrbuch deutscher Städte*. Statistical publications of the states of Prussia and Bavaria provided additional data to fill gaps in the data set. In addition, the *Medizinal-statistische Mitteilungen* of the Imperial Health Office and *Preussische Statistik* were also used. Particular care was taken in the collection of data on diarrhoeal disease, since the practice in Prussia differed markedly from the classification of disease used elsewhere. See Kintner, 'Determinants'.

[27]   Most of the data on temperatures is found in the *Statistisches Jahrbuch*. The *Statistisches Jahrbuch des deutschen Reiches* and H. Helm Clayton, *World Weather Records* (Washington, DC, 1927) provided additional data on temperature.

[28]   The sources include Kintner, 'Trends'; C. Röse, 'Die Wichtigkeit der Mutterbrust für die körperliche und geistige Entwicklung des Menschen', *Deutsche Monatsschrift für Zahnheilkunde*, 23 (1905), pp. 129–76; A. Bluhm, 'Stillhäufigkeit und Stilldauer', in A. Grotjahn and J. Kaup (eds), *Handwörterbuch der sozialen Hygiene* (Leipzig, 1912) and M.

legitimate and illegitimate fertility were calculated as the number of legitimate and illegitimate births per women aged fifteen to fifty. The absence of data on the marital status of the population for the entire sample precluded using marital and non-marital fertility rates. In addition, the share of stillbirths was included to account for the potential influence of neonatal mortality on infant mortality overall.

Finally, variables for policies that may have influenced the level of infant mortality were included. Some discussions of infant mortality have emphasised a potential link between water quality and diarrhoeal disease. For sanitation, they included the share of population that could be potentially served by a flush toilet and the share of property supplied with ground or spring water, or water from an impoundment. These sources of water were usually of superior quality to the filtered and unfiltered surface water from rivers and lakes used in many cities.[29] Dummy variables were used to indicate the presence of a milk dispensary and/or an infant welfare centre.[30] Table 10.3 provides the definition and the descriptive statistics for the independent variables used in the analysis. The statistics are presented for the full time series cross-section sample used in the estimation of the infant mortality relationship.

Following the practice in other statistical analyses of infant mortality, the dependent variable in each case was transformed as the log of the ratio of odds of the mortality event occurring. This transformation ensured that predictions would take on meaningful values by excluding the possibility of negative mortality. In addition, the logistic specification allows for ready interpretation of the quantitative impact of the estimated coefficients. Since Hausman tests rejected the presence of simultaneity bias, the equations for all four dependent variables – legitimate infant mortality, illegitimate infant mortality, infant mortality from diarrhoeal disease, and infant mortality from other causes – were estimated using Generalised Equation Estimation techniques for panel data. To remove any other spurious correlation, the lagged value of fertility was used. The specification included a random effect for each city and used an estimation of a robust variance-covariance matrix that was clustered on each city in the sample.

Groth, 'Die Säuglingsverhältnisse in Bayern', *Zeitschrift des bayerischen statistischen Landesamts*, 17 (1910), 78–164.

[29]   See *Statistisches Jahrbuch Deutscher Städte*, various issues. E. Grahn, *Die städtische Wasserversorgung im Deutschen Reiche sowie in einigen Nachbarländern* (Munich and Berlin, 1898 and 1902) and H. Salomon, *Die städtische Abwasserbeseitigung in Deutschland*, vols 1–3 (Jena, 1906).

[30]   See *Statistisches Jahrbuch deutscher Städte*; Tugendreich, 'Öffentliches Kinderschutz'; A. Keller, 'Der Umfang der Unterstützungen an stillende Mütter', *Zeitschrift für Säuglingsschutz*, 1 (1909), 180–85; *idem*, 'Sozial-hygienische Einrichtungen: Deutschland', A. Keller and C. Klunker (eds), *Säuglingsfürsorge und Kinderschutz in den europäischen Staaten, Part 1* (Berlin, 1912) and 'Berichten auf den Runderlass'.

Table 10.3: Descriptive statistics of variables used in the analysis

Independent variable	Mean	Standard deviation
No breastfeeding: share	0.243	0.089
Illegitimate fertility: births to unmarried women per all women aged 15–50 in previous year	0.013	0.006
Legitimate fertility: births to married women per all women aged 15–50 in previous year	0.100	0.030
Still births: per total births	0.032	0.006
Illegitimate births: share of total births	0.122	0.057
Water closets: share of population	0.452	0.454
Piped ground water: share of homes	0.689	0.407
Milk dispensary	0.263	0.440
Infant welfare centre	0.273	0.446
Summer temperature: average June to August (in degrees Celsius)	17.240	1.210
Share of employment in textiles	0.042	0.080
Share of employment in mining or metals	0.027	0.082

Results of the statistical analysis

Tables 10.4 and 10.5 present the results of the statistical analysis. The standardised coefficients provide a way of comparing the impact of each independent variable across the different regressions in explaining intra-sample variation in mortality rates. The larger the coefficient, the greater its impact on infant mortality. Consider the results for the mortality of legitimate infants. During this period, over five-sixths of all births were legitimate. The equation for 1889–1912 works well. It explains about one-half of the variance in infant mortality. The coefficients on the independent variables generally conform to the expected sign. A closer look at the relative magnitude of the standardised coefficients suggests that general fertility was the most important influence, followed by the degree to which mothers did not breastfeed their infants, the impact of the summer temperature, the availability of clean piped water, and the availability of water closets. The impact of greater resources available to the family, either through employment in the high-wage metal and coal sectors or through higher real wages, came close to the estimated importance of breastfeeding.

Table 10.4: The statistical analysis of the decline in infant mortality, 1889–1912

Independent variable	Legitimate		Illegitimate	
	Coefficient	Standardised coefficient	Coefficient	Standardised coefficient
No breastfeeding	0.88 (3.78)	0.25	0.27 (0.89)	0.07
Fertility	5.20 (7.73)	0.53	23.10 (2.22)	0.40
Still births	0.03 (1.75)	0.07	0.01 (0.35)	0.02
Illegitimate birth share			-0.06 (4.58)	-1.11
Water closets	-0.09 (2.49)	-0.11	-0.07 (1.04)	-0.08
Piped ground water	-0.10 (3.13)	-0.13	-0.15 (3.65)	-0.18
Milk dispensary	-0.10 (4.21)	-0.07	-0.16 (3.59)	-0.10
Infant welfare centre	-0.12 (5.14)	-0.07	-0.21 (4.24)	-0.10
Summer temperature	0.07 (9.85)	0.28	0.07 (7.60)	0.25
Textiles employment	0.10 (0.37)	0.03	0.31 (1.17)	0.08
Mining or metals employment	-1.06 (3.42)	-0.17	-0.82 (1.51)	-0.11
Female real wage	-0.13 (3.18)	-0.17	-0.14 (1.83)	-0.16
Constant	-3.07 (17.8)		-1.07 (4.35)	

Independent variable	Legitimate		Illegitimate	
	Coefficient	Standardised coefficient	Coefficient	Standardised coefficient
Test of model ($\div^2$)	718		368	
R^2	0.49		.41	
Mean of dependent variable	0.18		0.33	
N	1046		1041	

Source: Results of general estimating equation (GEE) regression analysis with random effects. Standard errors are corrected for hetereoskedasticity using White's matrix.
Notes: Absolute values of asymptotic *t*-statistics are in parentheses. The dependent variable is the logistic transformation of illegitimate and legitimate infant mortality.

Table 10.5: The statistical analysis of the decline in infant mortality from diarrhoeal and other causes, 1903–1912

Independent variable	Diarrhoeal disease		Other causes of death	
	Coefficient	Standardised coefficient	Coefficient	Standardised coefficient
No breastfeeding	0.72701 (1.87)	0.12	-0.04 (0.21)	-0.01
Illegitimate fertility	23.19 (3.12)	0.23	14.79 (3.98)	0.31
Legitimate fertility	9.99 (5.70)	0.64	2.56 (2.39)	0.31
Still births			0.02 (1.07)	0.05
Water closets	-0.18 (2.25)	-0.15	-0.01 (0.10)	-0.01
Piped ground water	-0.12 (0.98)	-0.10	-0.10 (2.21)	-0.16
Milk dispensary	-0.05 (1.03)	-0.05	-0.08 (2.83)	-0.15

Independent variable	Diarrhoeal disease		Other causes of death	
	Coefficient	Standardised coefficient	Coefficient	Standardised coefficient
Infant welfare centre	-0.12 (2.24)	-0.11	-0.07 (2.50)	-0.13
Summer temperature	0.15 (10.25)	0.38	0.02 (2.39)	0.09
Textiles employment	-0.63 (1.24)	-0.10	0.32 (0.93)	0.10
Mining or metals employment	-2.39 (3.79)	-0.51	-0.42 (1.10)	-0.18
Female real wage	-0.17 (1.74)	-0.11	-0.06 (1.03)	-0.08
Constant	-6.02 (5.58)		-2.64 (12.80)	
Test of model ($\div^2$)	231.1		94.9	
R^2	0.390		0.260	
Mean of dependent variable	0.065		0.107	
N	443		443	

Source: Results of general estimating equation (GEE) regression analysis with random effects. Standard errors are corrected for hetereoskedasticity using White's matrix.
Notes: Absolute values of asymptotic *t*-statistics are in parentheses. The dependent variable is the logistic transformation of infant mortality from diarrhoeal disease and infant mortality from other causes.

A comparison of the results for diarrhoeal disease in Table 10.5, with the results for legitimate infant mortality, suggests some important similarities. The regressions for diarrhoeal disease explained over two-fifths of the variance in mortality, while those for legitimate mortality explained about one-half. The standardised coefficients suggest that the variables capturing municipal interventions – water closets, piped ground water and infant welfare centres –

generally had influences of a similar magnitude.[31] As may be expected, water closets were much more important in explaining reductions in mortality from diarrhoeal disease than in the mortality of legitimate infants. High summer temperatures were substantially more important in explaining differences in mortality from diarrhoeal disease than the mortality of legitimate infants overall, or even mortality from other causes. This result is consistent with the medical literature of the time that emphasised the importance of diarrhoeal disease in explaining the summer peaks in mortality. Legitimate fertility was also much more important for causing mortality from diarrhoeal disease than mortality from other sources. Two important surprises point to other potential influences on infant diarrhoea than the feeding practices emphasised by the contemporary literature. Although designed to provide clean milk to weaned children, milk dispensaries had a negligible impact on diarrhoeal disease mortality. The absence of breastfeeding actually had a much weaker influence on mortality from diarrhoeal disease than on legitimate mortality overall; its influence on mortality from other causes was zero. Finally, the economic variables generally played a more important role in explaining diarrhoeal disease mortality than in explaining infant mortality overall. The high wages that resulted from employment in mining and metals sharply reduced infant mortality from diarrhoeal disease. A higher real wage for female day-labourers and a higher share of employment in textiles also reduced mortality from diarrhoeal disease. From these results, it is apparent that the improved conditions for raising infants that women could buy with higher income (either their own or the income of their husbands) more than offset the adverse effect of the reduction in time women had available to care for infants. In other words, the income effect most likely outweighed the substitution effect.

By comparison, although other causes of death (primarily respiratory illness and weakness of the infant at birth) accounted for almost two-thirds of infant mortality, the regression results presented in the fourth column of Table 10.5 are weaker than the results for diarrhoeal disease. The variables explain only one-quarter of the variation in infant mortality from other causes and the $\div^2$ statistic is much smaller. The influence of legitimate fertility within the sample was weaker, and the absence of breastfeeding had virtually no influence. High summer temperatures modestly increased mortality even though diseases such as respiratory infections were most often correlated with cold winter temperatures. This result may have stemmed from an indirect effect. Higher rates of morbidity from diarrhoeal disease may have weakened the resistance of the infant. The role of public intervention in reducing infant mortality from

---

[31]   It should be noted, however, that the size of the coefficients on 'Milk dispensary' and 'Infant welfare centre' is most likely overstated because of a spurious correlation. The spread of these services coincided almost exactly with the decline in infant mortality, and the influence of these services can be smaller when looking at cross-sectional evidence.

other causes of death also warrants mention. Water closets, as may be expected, had a minimal impact although clean water was relatively more important. Despite their focus, infant welfare centres and milk dispensaries had a stronger influence on this kind of mortality than on the mortality from diarrhoeal disease.

Finally, consider the results for illegitimate infant mortality. All told, deaths of infants of single mothers accounted for one-fifth of infant deaths in the larger German cities before the First World War. Of the various independent influences, the most important was the share of births out of wedlock. The higher share, the lower the risk of mortality to the infant, since the birth was more likely to occur to a woman who would subsequently get married to the father of the child and have adequate resources to raise the infant. Higher fertility had a similar impact as with legitimate births. What is perhaps most striking is the minimal influence of breastfeeding practices. It could be that the variable is poorly measured for unwed mothers, since high summer temperature explained about the same amount of differences in illegitimate infant mortality as in legitimate mortality. Provision of clean milk and infant welfare services were also rather more important than in the case of legitimate births. The economic variables played an equivalent role in explaining differences in mortality, although improved employment opportunities for women in the textile sector raised the likelihood of infant mortality.

Table 10.6: Predicted impacts of changes in important variables on infant mortality

Variable	Change	Predicted impact on deaths per 100 births			
		Legitimate	Illegitimate	Diarrhoeal	Other
No breastfeeding	Lower by 20%	-2.49	-5.44	-0.80	-0.07
Illegitimate fertility	Decr. by 0.1 births per 100		0.49	-0.13	-0.14
Legitimate fertility	Decr. by 2.2 births per 100	-1.62		-1.28	-0.55

		Legitimate	Illegitimate	Diarrhoeal	Other
Water closets	Install in entire city	-1.20	-1.50	-1.00	-0.05
Ground water	Provide to entire city	-1.50	-3.30	-0.70	-1.00
Milk dispensary	Establish in city	-1.40	-3.30	-0.29	-0.77
Infant health centre	Establish in city	-1.70	-4.40	-0.68	-0.64
Female real wage	Increase by 50 pfennig	-1.00	-1.49	-0.49	-0.29
Summer temperature	Increase by one degree	1.36	1.47	0.85	0.17
Actual decline		-8.5	-15.0	-2.9	-3.0

Source: Results of regression analysis.
Notes: The estimates for milk dispensaries and infant health centres are most likely too high. See discussion in text.

The statistical results provide an overview of the potential effectiveness of various measures in combating high infant mortality in Germany's larger cities. Table 10.6 summarises the impact of the kinds of changes in household behaviour and policy that may have reduced infant mortality. Most of the turn-of-the century efforts to combat infant mortality focused on policies to increase breastfeeding. In principle, these strategies could have had some impact, but their effectiveness may have been limited to the cities of southern Germany where large numbers of infants were never breastfed. Reducing the share of mothers never breastfeeding from one-fifth to one-twentieth of the population could have reduced mortality overall by 2.5 to 5.4 deaths per 100 births. This result is consistent with the widespread belief that single mothers were much less likely to breastfeed their infants, and it also underscores the focus of prevention efforts aimed at them. The estimated impact on diarrhoeal disease would be slightly under one less infant death per 100 births, a finding that seems low given the overwhelming emphasis in the contemporary literature on the importance of infant feeding practices for mortality from diarrhoea. The impact on mortality from other causes was zero. The most important change in household decision-making after 1900, which could have driven the decline in infant mortality, was the fall in fertility of about one-quarter by 1912. The estimated impact of this decline would account for about one-fifth of the actual reduction in infant mortality. This result is a fraction of three-quarters resulting from Kintner's regression analysis of substantially aggregated data over a longer time frame. The impact of a decline would have been much more important for a reduction in illegitimate infant mortality, but illegitimate births actually increased about 10 per cent from the 1880s to 1912. This prompted a modest increase in illegitimate infant mortality.

The policies designed to achieve the goal of reducing infant mortality would appear to have had only a limited effectiveness. A full program of milk dispensaries and infant health centres would imply at most a predicted decline of 3.1 in legitimate infant mortality, but a drop of only 0.9 in mortality from diarrhoeal disease. As noted above, these estimates most likely overestimate the impact of these measures because of the confounding influence of the general decline in infant mortality in the decade before the First World War. These measures would be much more effective in reducing the mortality of infants born to single mothers. In addition, they would have a stronger influence on other causes of infant death from 1903 on. Both of these results suggest that these programs were potentially more effective as providers of income transfers and direct care to the poorest and most vulnerable mothers and infants rather than providing mothers with new information about infant feeding practices.

A full program of sanitary improvement appears to have had the potential of reducing infant mortality to all mothers, including the poorest single mothers. As would be expected, the impact of sanitary improvement on mortality from diarrhoeal disease was much stronger than on mortality from other causes. Of course, the proportional reduction would been much stronger since diarrhoeal disease accounted for only about two-fifths of infant deaths. This result is also at variance with Kintner's conclusions, which were based on much more aggregated analysis.

It is worthwhile noting how critical the impact of higher summer temperatures was for influencing short-term changes in infant mortality. An increase in the average summer temperature from the long-run average of about 17 degrees to the 19 degrees that prevailed during 1911 in these cities, would increase mortality from all causes an estimated 2.7 deaths per 100 live births, or an amount sufficient to offset all of the benefits of sanitary reform. Deaths from diarrhoeal disease would rise by 1.7 per 100, or one-quarter above the mortality rate prevailing in the early 1900s.

Conclusion

This analysis of infant mortality decline before the First World War suggests that casting the problem as one of household choice can provide insights into some of the causal links and potential statistical biases that may otherwise be missing from an analysis based primarily upon an epidemiological approach. Once the potential behavioural links have been clarified, it is then possible to assess questions such as the effectiveness of public intervention as it attempted to modify both local environments and behaviour. The statistical analysis that emerges from such an approach suggests that the classic public health measures of providing clean water and finding effective methods of removing human waste could have contributed to the decline in infant mortality as well. In the case of German cities, although sewers and piped water were available to most residents by the turn of the century, the changeover to flush toilets occurred somewhat later. The particularly high density of German housing, with the attendant widespread sharing of toilet facilities, meant that the risk of transmission of diarrhoeal disease was heightened. Other measures of the infant welfare movement could have been effective to the extent that they provided assistance in improved care and better resources for the poorest mothers.

The focus of the German infant welfare movement on increasing rates of breastfeeding appears to have been rather off the mark. Poverty, particularly of single mothers, and poor sanitary provision and practices appear to have been at least as important as inadequate breastfeeding. Of course, the data available to us today from this period are most likely inadequate to the task of directly testing this hunch. One approach that could help would be a closer look at the underlying aetiology of infant diarrhoeal diseases at the turn of the century in order to verify whether the faecal–oral path of transmission played the role that this analysis implies. In addition, a more careful appraisal of household decision-making is needed in order to better gauge the actual effectiveness of public health measures.

11

Decline of the urban penalty: milk supply and infant welfare centres in Germany, 1890s to 1920s

Jörg Peter Vögele, Wolfgang Woelk and Silke Fehlemann

The urban penalty

Cities in historical Europe were unhealthy.[1] Urbanisation and industrialisation radically changed living conditions and took their toll on the inhabitants. Terms like 'urban graveyard' or 'urban penalty' emphasised the high death rates found in the rapidly-growing towns of nineteenth-century Europe: rates which significantly exceeded the average for rural areas or the whole country.[2] Detailed research charting the demographic transition has been undertaken for England and Wales, Sweden and more recently for Germany.[3] Towards the end of the nineteenth century, urban mortality rates in several Western European countries improved substantially, both in relative and in absolute terms. The gap between urban and rural mortality narrowed as a consequence and the 'urban penalty', which had been generally evident throughout Europe in earlier decades, was attenuated or disappeared entirely.[4] In this context, recent research has emphasised the interrelationship between urbanisation and population development during the demographic and epidemiological transitions, and has suggested that the effect of public health provision on the secular decline in urban mortality has been underestimated.[5]

---

[1] See for example A.F. Weber, *The Growth of the Cities in the Nineteenth Century. A Study in Statistics* (New York, 1899).

[2] G. Kearns, 'The Urban Penalty and the Population History of England', in A. Brändström and L. Tedebrand (eds), *Society, Health and Population during the Demographic Transition* (Stockholm, 1988), pp. 213–36.

[3] R. Woods and J. Woodward (eds), *Urban Disease and Mortality in Nineteenth Century England* (London, 1984).

[4] J. Vögele, *Urban Mortality Change in England and Germany, 1870–1910* (Liverpool, 1998).

[5] Woods and Woodward, *Urban Disease*; Kearns, 'Urban Penalty'; G. Kearns, 'Le handicap urbain et le déclin de la mortalité en Angleterre et au Pays de Galles 1851–1900',

Urbanisation is understood as a quantitative process of population growth. In 1871, 36 per cent of the German population lived in communities of 2,000 or more inhabitants; by 1910 the proportion was 60 per cent: one-fifth of the population was concentrated in big cities of more than 100,000 inhabitants.[6] This process was accompanied initially by rising death rates. Urban death rates in Germany reached their peak after the middle of the nineteenth century. Thereafter, urban mortality improved. An epidemiological analysis gives further insights into the mechanisms of this decline and in this chapter the urban disease profile is reconstructed, using data from the ten largest towns. As there is no corresponding data available for rural areas or the national aggregate, Prussian regional data will be used as a basis for comparison.[7] After discussion of the changing disease profile and its effects on the urban penalty, two examples, milk supply and the creation of infant welfare centres, will be used to provide an analysis of public health measures introduced as attempts to improve health in the cities of imperial Germany.

The urban disease profile

In Germany the urban disease profile (indicated by the sample of ten towns) was initially dominated by the gastrointestinal diseases, which almost exclusively affected infants. In the 1870s, more than one-third of all deaths could be attributed to gastrointestinal disorders (including diarrhoea and convulsions). The second main killer was the respiratory disease complex (including tuberculosis) responsible for slightly more than one-fifth of all deaths. These were followed by 'other causes' (134/1,000 deaths), diseases of the brain and nerves (82/1,000 deaths), childhood infectious diseases, including diphtheria and measles (78/1,000 deaths), degenerative diseases, such as cancer and diseases of the heart and circulatory system (62/1,000 deaths) and infirmity (45/1,000 deaths). The classic infectious diseases, for example smallpox, were

Annales de Démographie Historique (1993), 75–105; G. Kearns, W.R. Lee and J. Rogers, 'The Interactions of Political and Economic Factors in the Management of Urban Public Health', in M.C. Nelson and J. Rogers (eds), *Urbanisation and the Epidemiologic Transition* (Uppsala, 1989), pp. 9–81; S. Szreter, 'The Importance of Social Intervention in Britain's Mortality Decline 1850–1914, a Reinterpretation of the Role of Public Health', *Social History of Medicine*, 1 (1988), 1–37. Similar conclusions were reached for France. See S.H. Preston and E. van de Walle, 'Urban French Mortality in the Nineteenth Century', *Population Studies*, 32 (1978), 275–97.

[6]   G. Hohorst, J. Kocka and G.A. Ritter (eds), *Sozialgeschichtliches Arbeitsbuch. Materialien zur Statistik des Kaiserreichs 1870–1914* (Munich, 1975), p. 43.

[7]   For a systematic comparison of urban and rural Prussia see J. Vögele, 'Différences entre ville et campagne et évolution de la mortalité en Allemagne pendant l'industrialisation', *Annales de Démographie Historique*, 1996, 249–68.

no longer of epidemiological importance; others, like cholera, had only local or regional impact.

After the turn of the century the urban disease profile altered. The incidence of gastrointestinal diseases (260/1,000 deaths) was reduced to the same level as respiratory diseases (260/1,000 deaths), followed by degenerative diseases (173/1,000 deaths), 'other causes' (146/1,000 deaths), diseases of the brain and nervous system (75/1,000 deaths), childhood infectious diseases (53/1,000 deaths) and infirmity (33/1,000 deaths). When compared to the Prussian disease profile, most of the diseases showed higher death rates in the urban context (Table 11.1). The gastrointestinal diseases were responsible for the higher overall death rates in urban areas, followed by respiratory diseases. In contrast, death rates from childhood infectious diseases were lower in urban areas, when compared to the aggregate figures of Prussia for 1877. Similarly, the death rate for infirmity was also lower in urban areas. The higher rate in Prussia might be the result of a bias in diagnosis. In the absence of obligatory official certification of cause of death by medical personnel in Prussia and a low doctor–patient ratio in rural areas, relatives of the deceased regularly 'diagnosed' infirmity.

By 1907 the picture had changed again in some crucial respects. Overall mortality was lower in the sample of German towns when compared to Prussia. The urban advantage in the childhood disease complex had disappeared, and there was a substantial reduction of the urban penalty with respect to mortality from gastrointestinal and respiratory diseases and much lower death rates from 'other causes'. The latter might be due to changes in the Prussian cause-of-death registration system in 1904, when convulsions (formerly in the gastrointestinal diseases category) were grouped among 'other causes', whereas the cities, with their own statistical offices, still counted them amongst the gastrointestinal diseases.[8] This implies that, with respect to gastrointestinal disease, the reduction of the urban penalty was even more pronounced. The contribution of various diseases to the overall urban mortality decline was distributed differentially (Table 11.1). In the German towns, gastrointestinal diseases played a disproportionate role in the urban mortality decline between 1877 and 1907, contributing 56 per cent of the total, followed by the respiratory disease complex accounting for 19 per cent. The overall decline in urban mortality was substantially counterbalanced by an increase in deaths from degenerative diseases of 13 per cent.

---

[8]   'Preußen. Erlaß, betr. die Neubearbeitung des Verzeichnisses der Krankheiten und Todesursachen', *Veröffentlichungen des Kaiserlichen Gesundheitsamtes*, 28 (1904), pp. 645–51; *Preußische Statistik*, 189 (1905), p. 6. See also H.J. Kintner, 'Classifying Causes of Death during the Late Nineteenth and Early Twentieth Centuries: The Case of German Infant Mortality', *Historical Methods*, 19, 2 (1986), 47.

Table 11.1: Cause-specific mortality change in the largest German towns

Cause of death	SMR* (per 10,000 living)		Decline 1877–1907		Differentials towns/Prussia	
	1877	1907	Absolute	Relative	1877	1907
Childhood infectious diseases	23	10	13	12	-13	0
Gastrointestinal diseases	106	48	58	56	30	9
Respiratory diseases	68	48	20	19	19	4
Degenerative diseases	18	32	-14	-13	6	11
Brain and nerves	24	14	10	9	9	3
Infirmity	13	6	6	6	-13	-12
Other causes	39	27	12	11	-3	-18
All causes	290	184	107	100	35	-3

* – standardised on the population structure of Prussia 1877.
Sources: Statistical yearbooks of selected towns and states.

Changes in the incidence of gastrointestinal diseases formed a major element in explaining both the urban–rural divide and the urban mortality decline in Germany. In particular, the gastrointestinal diseases affected infant death rates, peaking in the hot summer months. In 1877, almost 87 per cent of all deaths from gastrointestinal diseases in the largest German towns occurred amongst infants. This represented 63 per cent of all infant deaths for that year. In 1907 the figures were a little lower: 78 per cent of all deaths from gastrointestinal diseases were infants, some 60 per cent of all infant deaths. The level and trend of mortality from gastrointestinal diseases was therefore closely linked to overall infant mortality rates. As the source material for infant mortality is less problematic, the discussion will now focus on urban infant mortality rates.

Urban infant mortality rates significantly surpassed those in rural areas at the beginning of our period, but urban rates declined from their high level at the beginning of the registration period. In contrast, the decline for rural Prussia did not begin before the first decades of the twentieth century (Figure 11.1). During the course of the twentieth century towns showed increasingly lower infant mortality rates than the rural areas, or indeed, the national aggregate.[9] Key explanatory factors, cited in recent studies as determining levels and trends of infant mortality, include legitimacy status of infants, fertility, feeding

---

9   Source: *Preußische Statistik*.

practices, housing conditions, parental education, wealth and occupation.[10] For Germany, levels and trends of infant mortality, as well as social and regional variations, have already been discussed in detail. Regional differences in infant mortality have been attributed, to a large extent, to different attitudes towards life and death.[11] In Prussia during the late nineteenth century, however, regional disparities were diminishing, whereas social differentials increased.[12] As these were not identical with class formation, mortality change cannot be exclusively

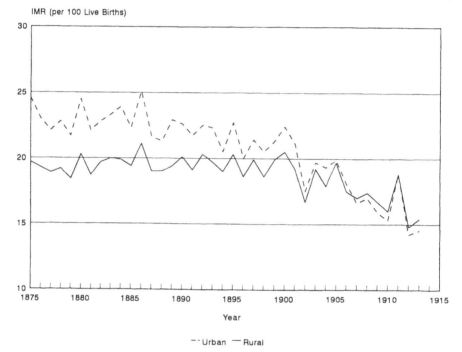

Figure 11.1: Infant mortality in Prussia 1877–1913

---

[10] R. Woods, P.A. Watterson and J.H. Woodward, 'The Causes of Rapid Infant Mortality Decline in England and Wales', *Population Studies*, 42 (1988), 343–66; 43 (1989), 113–32.

[11] A.E. Imhof, 'Unterschiedliche Säuglingsterblichkeit in Deutschland, 18. bis 20. Jahrhundert – Warum?', *Zeitschrift für Bevölkerungswissenschaft*, 7, 3 (1981), 343–82. See also U. Ottmüller, 'Speikinder-Gedeihkinder: Kommunikationstheoretische Überlegungen zu Gestalt und Funktion frükindlicher Sozialisation im bäuerlichen Lebenszusammenhang des deutschsprachigen 19. und frühen 20. Jahrhunderts' (unpublished PhD thesis, University of Berlin, 1986).

[12] R. Spree, *Health and Social Class in Imperial Germany. A Social Study of Mortality, Morbidity and Inequality* (Oxford, 1988); *idem, On Infant Mortality Change in Germany since the Early Nineteenth Century* (Münchener Wirtschaftswissenschaftliche Beiträge, Nr. 95–03) (Munich, 1995).

explained in terms of differences in wealth. On the contrary, feeding practices have been identified as a major component of the high infant mortality rates in nineteenth-century Germany.[13]

In this context, however, it is of special importance that the decline in urban infant mortality occurred at the same time as the traditionally low breastfeeding rates declined at an increasing rate. In view of this development, public health measures aiming at environmental improvements and later at infants, as a particular 'at-risk' group, might have played a more important role in determining urban mortality change.[14] During the last quarter of the nineteenth century, the cities developed new public health strategies that attacked the problems of urban health at several levels. The big cities, in particular, possessed the potential to introduce a variety of public health measures and therefore played an important and active part in the struggle against disease and epidemics as well as in the development of modern public health strategies. Urban spaces represented more than large conglomerations of people that were inherently unhealthy: there were advantages as well as disadvantages.

Public health and the urban mortality decline

Specific public health measures were carried out in an increasingly systematic manner during the late nineteenth and the early twentieth centuries. Sanitary reform focused on measures that were intended to improve the hygienic conditions of the urban environment. Particular emphasis was first placed on central water supplies and sewerage systems and other services included street cleansing and waste disposal.[15] Towards the end of the nineteenth century, attention shifted from environmental measures towards the protection of at-risk urban groups. A major element of these strategies became the fight against high infant mortality. Special emphasis was placed on municipal milk supply and infant welfare campaigns. Whereas high infant mortality was traditionally considered a matter of fate, which could not be averted, decreasing birth rates towards the end of the nineteenth century, prompted fears that Germany's future would be at risk from an economic and military point of view. The direct comparisons with England and France triggered hectic activities in industry and politics. Municipal milk supply became a high priority and, after the turn of the

---

[13]   H. J. Kintner, 'The Determinants of Infant Mortality in Germany from 1871 to 1933' (unpublished PhD thesis, University of Michigan, 1982); S. Stöckel, 'Säuglingssterblichkeit in Berlin von 1870 bis zum Vorabend des ersten Weltkriegs – Eine Kurve mit hohem Maximum und starkem Gefälle', *Berlin-Forschungen*, 1 (1986), 219–64.

[14]   See J. Vögele, 'Urban Infant Mortality in Imperial Germany', *Social History of Medicine*, 7 (1994), 414–20.

[15]   T. Weyl, 'Assanierung', in T. Weyl (ed.), *Soziale Hygiene. Handbuch der Hygiene*, 4. Supplement-Band (Jena, 1904), p. 1.

century, infant welfare centres were created with the aim of raising low breastfeeding rates. However, infant welfare policies were initially restricted to aspects of nutrition with little consideration of socio-political measures.[16]

The supply of adequate milk was considered a central municipal responsibility. This involved using the available technical treatments of animal milk – pasteurisation and sterilisation – according to contemporary scientific standards. During the late 1880s, the distribution of treated milk was initiated. Taking the French example of the Goutte-de-Lait-Movement, municipal milk depots were opened in Germany from the 1890s onwards. The number of depots reached its peak in 1913: in 85 towns there were 258 retail stores with a total turnover of 4.93 million litres per year. These figures are not as impressive as they might seem. This turnover is equivalent to the amount needed as an adequate supply for the whole of Düsseldorf for a period of six weeks.[17] The urban milk supply was originally handled by private traders, but local communities gradually tried to set up their own systems of supply and distribution for various reasons.[18] First, the communities aimed at achieving better control of the urban milk trade; second, the municipal authorities wanted to supply good-quality milk at a favourable price to those inhabitants who needed it most. During periods of crisis and war the daily supply of milk could not be guaranteed. In March 1913, 134,000 litres of milk were supplied daily in Düsseldorf (a peak rate which was only reached again at the end of the 1920s). During the First World War the amount of milk available each day rapidly decreased. In October 1915, 68,500 litres were supplied. In December 1916, this had declined to 36,000 litres and by February 1919 there were only 11,000 litres. In June 1919 still only 20,000 litres were available.[19]

The regulation of milk did not come under the Imperial Foodstuffs Regulations and by 1900 only three cities (Berlin, Dresden and Munich) had imposed special municipal regulations on milk for infants. It is not surprising, therefore, that there were extensive contemporary complaints about the poor quality of the milk.[20] In 1910, the Düsseldorf journalist Isaak Thalheimer

---

[16] U. Frevert, 'The Civilizing Tendency of Hygiene. Working-Class Women under Medical Control in Imperial Germany', in J.C. Fout (ed.), *German Women in the Nineteenth Century. A Social History* (New York, 1984), pp. 320–44.

[17] *Die deutsche Milchwirtschaft in Wort und Bild*. Redigiert von Kurt Friedel und Prof. Dr Arthur Keller (Halle, 1914), p. xix. W. Woelk, 'Der Düsseldorfer Milchkrieg. Ein Beitrag zur Sozial geschichte der Ernahrung im fruhen 20. Jahrhundert', im *Dusseldorfer Jahrbuch*, 69 (1998), 211–35.

[18] L. Spiegel, 'Kommunale Milchversorgung', *Schriften des Vereins für Socialpolitik*, 128 (1908), p. 232.

[19] *Statistische Jahresberichte der Stadt Düsseldorf.*

[20] C. Flügge, 'Die Aufgaben und Leistungen der Milchsterilisierung gegenüber den Darmkrankheiten der Säuglinge', *Zeitschrift für Hygiene und Infectionskrankheiten*, 17 (1894), p. 321.

investigated the adulteration of milk.[21] His report mentioned court verdicts against corrupt traders whose sampled milk was diluted and had shown traces of faeces, straw and formaldehyde. Before 1901, police officers tested milk merely by its taste and smell. Milk that failed these subjective tests, conducted by untrained officers, was only the tip of the iceberg. However, after 1901, the milk and dairy trade in Düsseldorf was legally controlled. It was now possible to identify responsible traders, in the case of a complaint, as they were registered with the police authorities.[22] The milk the bona fide traders imported into the city had to be registered and inspected.

Although the percentage of contaminated milk in Düsseldorf found by laboratory tests decreased from 23 per cent in 1895 to 3 per cent in 1906,[23] the bacteriological investigations to determine the microbial content remained complicated and it was still hard to carry out tests on a daily basis.[24] This was one of the reasons why the amount of specially treated and controlled infant milk remained very low (a contemporary source mentioned a daily amount of 500 litres per 100,000 inhabitants). As the price of the controlled milk was 50 to 60 Pfennige per litre, over twice as much as the price of uncontrolled milk, it was only accessible to the wealthier middle classes and above.[25] The food industry was aware of the small amount of high-quality milk and tried to bring artificial substitutes for milk onto the market. This was done by expensive, large-scale publicity campaigns, allegedly supported by scientific experts. For example, in Bonn in 1902, young families automatically received an information brochure, signed by a paediatrician, recommending a particular brand of dried milk.[26]

A major cause of milk supply problems in the large cities was transportation. Dairy production within urban areas decreased continuously as industrialisation increased. Consequently, large amounts of milk had to be imported. The long distances and the lack of appropriate means of transportation from the production sites led to a significant deterioration in milk quality, especially during the hot summer months. The furthest dairy from Düsseldorf was 80 kilometres. Moreover, the milk was seldom completely sterilised, because this process was expensive. Despite these deficiencies, public health officials were convinced that the municipal milk supply was a successful undertaking and that it had a positive impact on infant mortality

[21]   I. Thalheimer, *Milchversorgung* (Düsseldorf, 1922, 5th edition), pp. 4–6.
[22]   F. Schrakamp, 'Gesundheitswesen', in T. Weyl (ed.), *Die Assanierung der Städte in Einzeldarstellungen, vol. 2.2: Die Assanierung von Düsseldorf* (Leipzig, 1908), 110–13.
[23]   Schrakamp, 'Gesundheitswesen', p. 110.
[24]   Pfaffenholz, 'Wichtige Aufgaben der öffentlichen und privaten Wohlfahrtspflege auf dem Gebiet der künstlichen Ernährung der Säuglinge', *Centralblatt für allgemeine Gesundheitspflege*, 21 (1902), 400.
[25]   Pfaffenholz, 'Aufgaben', 404.
[26]   Cramer, Contribution to the discussion following Pfaffenholz, 'Aufgaben', 419.

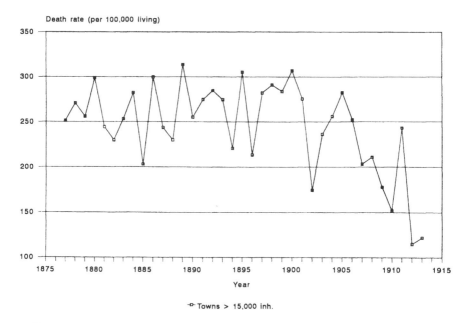

Figure 11.2: Acute digestive diseases: mortality 1877–1913 in German towns (per 10,000 living)

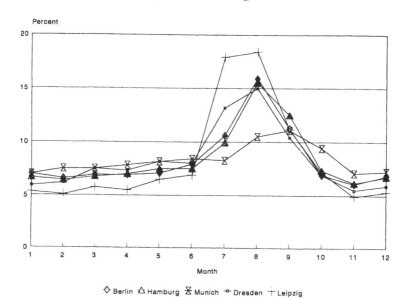

Figure 11.3: Seasonal distribution of infant mortality in selected cities, 1898–1902 (%)

rates. Technologies and a bureaucracy able to impose health regulations in their opinion counteracted the urban experience of being removed from the site of milk production.

Today scholars differ widely in their conclusions about the impact of milk supply on the course of infant mortality. Beaver and Dwork conclude that the substantial decrease in English infant mortality rates after the turn of the century was mainly a result of the improved supply of pasteurised milk.[27] More recent and methodologically stronger studies by Woods, Watterson and Woodward are sceptical about the influence of the municipal milk supply on the decrease in infant mortality in Britain. As breastfeeding remained widespread, the health of infants would have been more dependent on other demographic and socio-economic issues.[28] Atkins states that the frequent use of milk of inferior quality was the cause of general poor health.[29]

As breastfeeding rates were relatively low in Germany, the potential impact of municipal milk was of greater significance. Indeed, in towns with over 15,000 inhabitants the average death rates from gastrointestinal diseases showed a considerable decrease at the beginning of the twentieth century (Figure 11.2).[30] Nevertheless, variations in the weather continued to play some part. The cool summer of 1902 resulted in a low infant mortality rate, whereas the extremely hot summer of 1911 drastically increased infant mortality. The annual seasonal variations also persisted. Figure 11.3 shows the typical summer peak for the five large cities of Berlin, Hamburg, Munich, Dresden and Leipzig from 1898 until 1902.[31] According to investigations in Berlin, the infants who received milk substitutes were affected, whereas breastfeeding provided a certain protection during the hot summer months (Figure 11.4).[32] Not until the First World War did this summer peak diminish. In view of the poor state of the milk supply, especially during the years of the war, the flattening-out of the seasonal pattern was more likely the result of changing attitudes of mothers towards breastfeeding because of the poor economic situation. A long-term increase in breastfeeding rates continued into the 1920s. After the period from 1926 to 1928, the summer peak gradually disappeared in the five large cities mentioned above (Figure 11.5).[33]

[27]   M.W. Beaver, 'Population, Infant Mortality and Milk', *Population Studies*, 27 (1973), 243–54; D. Dwork, *War is Good for Babies and Other Young Children: A History of the Infant and Child Welfare Movement in England, 1898–1918* (London and New York, 1987).

[28]   Woods, Watterson and Woodward, 'Causes', 116–20.

[29]   P.J. Atkins, 'White Poison?: The Social Consequences of Milk Consumption in London, 1850–1939', *Social History of Medicine*, 5 (1992), 227.

[30]   *Veröffentlichungen des Kaiserlichen Gesundheitsamtes (Beilagen)*, 1878–1914.

[31]   F. Prinzing, *Handbuch der medizinischen Statistik* (Jena, 1930 [2]), p. 402.

[32]   *Statistisches Jahrbuch der Stadt Berlin*, 32 (1913), p. 183.

[33]   Prinzing, *Handbuch* (1930), p. 402.

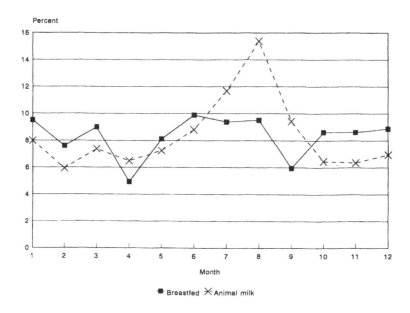

Figure 11.4: Seasonal distribution of infant mortality in Berlin (1908) according to feeding practices (%)

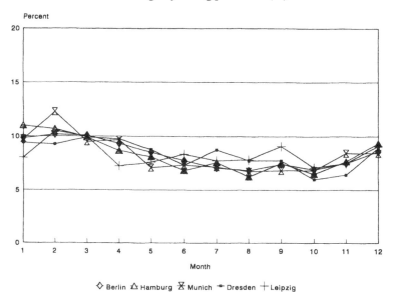

Figure 11.5: Seasonal distribution of infant mortality in selected cities, 1926–28 (%)

Infant welfare

While some contemporary observers regarded the improvement of the milk supply around the turn of the century as the best means of practical welfare work, after 1900 the idea was generally accepted that a broader range of measures must be implemented to combat high infant mortality rates. Better hygienic standards of milk; extensive infant welfare programmes (which included breastfeeding campaigns) and widespread education about possible causes of infant death were the major focuses of the many infant welfare societies founded in imperial Germany during the first decade of the twentieth century. After the call for intensification of infant welfare work by the Prussian Empress, Auguste Victoria, in November 1904, Düsseldorf was the first city to launch a new, comprehensive concept of infant welfare. This programme attempted to unite government, local communities and private welfare workers in the Society for Infant Welfare in the Administrative District of Düsseldorf.

The Society is an important example of the history of infant, child and youth health care. At first, as a regional association, it took a mediating role between state and local social politics. Moreover, its representatives formed a modern caring system in a region characterised by rapid industrialisation on the one hand, but also with large rural areas on the other. With its modern approach to welfare, the Society achieved a leading role in imperial Germany. Increasingly, the Society concentrated not only on infant care, but also expanded its activities towards child and youth welfare. With its innovative approach it shaped the form of public child and youth welfare in this region after the First World War.

The initiative for the Society's foundation lay in the hands of Arthur Schlossmann, the director of the Düsseldorf children's hospital. Schlossmann, born in 1867, had trained as a paediatrician in Berlin. When he moved to Dresden in the early 1890s, he founded a Policlinic for Infants and Children and became involved in a range of related initiatives. In 1906, he moved to the recently-founded Academy of Practical Medicine at Düsseldorf. His social-hygienic approach was based on stringent asepsis, natural methods and education.[34] For this purpose he proposed an integrated welfare service.[35] After negotiations with state and municipal officials (concerning finance), the Society was founded on 7 November 1907 with Schlossmann as chairman. All rural districts (*Landkreise*) and towns (*kreisfreie Städte*) of the administrative

---

[34]   P. Weindling, *Health, Race and German Politics between National Unification and Nazism, 1870–1945* (Cambridge, 1989), p. 202.

[35]   W. Woelk, 'Von der Gesundheitsfürsorge zur Wohlfahrtspflege: Gesundheitsfürsorge im rheinisch-westfälischen Industriegebiet am Beispiel des Vereins für Säuglingsfürsorge im Regierungsbezirk Düsseldorf', in J. Vögele and W. Woelk (eds), *Stadt, Krankheit und Tod. Geschichte der Städtischen Gesundheitsverhältnisse während der Epidemiologischen Transition* (Berlin, 2000), pp. 339–59.

area became founding members. Together they contributed an annual fee of 20,000 marks.[36] At the end of the first fiscal year, the Society had already grown to 350 members, including representatives of local businesses and associations. Individuals who held key positions as policy-makers or managers of the local economy also participated.[37] The Society was thus a combination of the relevant institutions, associations and individuals responsible for directing or influencing welfare policy in the region and was placed on a solid financial and political basis. In the second year Dr Marie Baum, a trained chemist and former factory inspector, was employed as chief executive, and the management became professionalised. Initially, the Society compiled information using a classification of the regional differences in infant mortality in the Düsseldorf district (Figure 11.6).[38] There was no clear urban penalty: infant mortality varied from 9.8 per cent in the south-eastern rural areas of the Bergisches Land to 19.9 per cent in the rural area of Neuss, which was as high as in the city of Düsseldorf.

As there was no clear urban penalty, the Society for Infant Welfare concentrated their efforts not only on the very industrialised cities in the Düsseldorf district, but also covered the rural areas in order to even out the spatial differences in infant mortality rates. It launched a wide range of activities that took into account the different economic structures and religious backgrounds and the varying population densities in the Düsseldorf area. The Society distributed leaflets and brochures, offered free medical advice and held regular courses in the towns of the area. In addition, two female teachers were employed to work in the rural areas. They used mobile equipment and moved from village to village. With illustrated material, photographs and even films they tried to demonstrate recent scientific knowledge, to explain the physical development of infants and to propagate adequate methods of infant care in a popular way. Mothers could obtain several welfare benefits. The Society offered breastfeeding rewards, which offered a limited amount of financial help. Furthermore, the mothers could potentially save an expensive doctor's visit if they attended the preventive check-ups offered for infants. During infant health-care courses, mothers were taught about raising infants and adopting a more hygienic lifestyle. In some welfare centres they could also receive quality cow's milk and infants' clothes.

---

[36]   A. Schlossmann, 'Über die Organisation des Vereins für Säuglingsfürsorge im Regierungsbezirke Düsseldorf', *Concordia. Zeitschrift der Zentralstelle für Volkswohlfahrt*, 15 (1908), 239–49.

[37]   *Bericht über das erste Geschäftsjahr des Vereins für Säuglingsfürsorge im Regierungsbezirk Düsseldorf 1907*, Appendix.

[38]   *Bericht über das zweite Geschäftsjahr des Vereins für Säuglingsfürsorge im Regierungsbezirk Düsseldorf 1908/09*, Anlage.

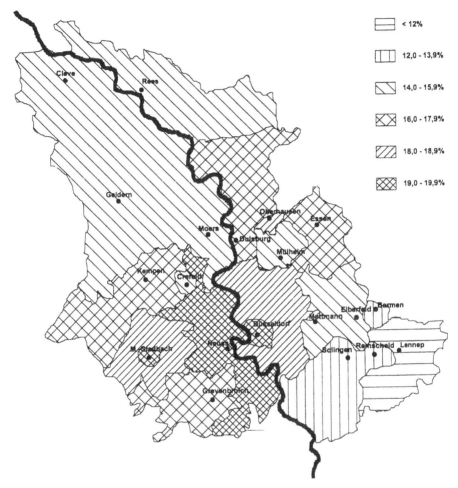

Figure 11.6: Infant mortality Regierungsbezirk Düsseldorf 1902–6

Source: Geschäftsbericht des Vereins für Säuglingsfürsorge 1907/8.

Most of the contemporary reformers were convinced of the success of these campaigns and many modern historians accept this view.[39] However, a comprehensive analysis of the acceptance and the effectiveness of the Society's activities might modify this picture. Such a reanalysis investigates how the target group was contacted, whether the mothers accepted the welfare workers voluntarily, what kind of welfare measures were successful and which could not reach the working-class mothers at all. For example, even in 1927 there were complaints that despite home visits and financial support for breastfeeding, many mothers could not be supported by the local advisory centres. The proud announcement that between 60 and 80 per cent of the mothers in a town were routinely contacted must be regarded with scepticism.[40] Medical experts involved in health visiting conceded that even in an industrial city such as Dortmund the rate did not surpass 60 or 70 per cent despite very substantial efforts.[41] Moreover, this refers to single visits and provides no indication of the intensity or frequency of the contacts.

Surveys from other areas reported even lower contact rates. In Leipzig, for example, out of 55,776 live births during the period 1907–10 only 3,301 infants, that is 5.9 per cent, came into contact with the campaigners.[42] Contemporary investigations of the impact of breastfeeding rewards are few and far between. Surveys taken at the centres in Berlin, Breslau, Cologne, Karlsruhe, Leipzig and Munich suggest that the campaigners' work raised neither the frequency nor the duration of breastfeeding substantially.[43] In Munich almost 90 per cent of all mothers who received breastfeeding rewards had already breastfed their previous babies, born before incentives were offered. Similarly, the duration of breastfeeding was not extended when compared to children born earlier.[44]

It is also important to distinguish between married and unmarried mothers when discussing acceptance. Reports about the visitors in advisory centres in the Düsseldorf region argued that married mothers accepted the welfare centres more willingly than unmarried mothers.[45] The distrust of unmarried mothers

---

[39]   See for example H. Brüchert-Schunk, *Städtische Sozialpolitik vom wilhelminischen Reich bis zur Weltwirtschaftskrise. Eine sozial- und kommunalhistorische Untersuchung am Beispiel der Stadt Mainz 1890–1930* (Stuttgart, 1994), pp. 181–6.

[40]   For a more optimistic view see Frevert, 'The Civilizing Tendency', pp. 320–44.

[41]   S. Engel and H. Behrendt, 'Säuglingsfürsorge', in A. Gottstein, A. Schlossmann and L. Teleky (eds), *Handbuch der Sozialen Hygiene*, vol. 4 (Berlin, 1927), p. 97.

[42]   H. Risel and F. Schmitz, 'Ueber Stillprämien und ihre Erfolge', *Archiv für Kinderheilkunde*, 59 (1913), 57.

[43]   F. Rott, *Umfang, Bedeutung und Ergebnisse der Unterstützungen an stillende Mütter* (Berlin, 1914), pp. 46–51.

[44]   Uffenheimer, 'Zwei Jahre offene Säuglingsfürsorge', *Münchener Medizinische Wochenschrift*, 58 (1911), 308–11; 361–4.

[45]   *Bericht über das fünfte Geschäftsjahr des Vereins für Säuglingsfürsorge im Regierungsbezirk Düsseldorf 1911/12*, p. 29.

resulted from the legal status of their children. Illegitimate children had to be kept under the care of an official guardian and state authorities possessed the right to put unmarried mothers under police supervision if they were suspected of neglecting their children. With the increase of welfare work, state control passed into the hands of trained female welfare workers, yet the deep mistrust of unmarried mothers persisted. A visit to the welfare centre could expose them to supervision, and therefore they tried to avoid any contact with the welfare workers. If a mother was suspected of neglecting her child, she could be compelled to visit the welfare centre or endure compulsory home visits.[46] Married mothers were obliged to regularly attend the welfare centres only if they received breastfeeding rewards. Although the organisers of breastfeeding support tried to avoid any connection to poor relief, in practice, however, mothers had to face long bureaucratic procedures with intimidating and discriminating investigations.[47]

Another crucial difference in the mothers' acceptance of welfare centres is related to the location of the centre. A higher acceptance of welfare centres was found in the larger cities of the district than in the rural areas. For example, in the city of Düsseldorf there were complaints about overcrowding during consultation hours. The municipal authorities responded by employing an additional physician.[48] In terms of the use of the Society's centres, despite their flaws, it appears that there was a rural rather than an urban penalty.

As another part of the practical welfare work, a home visiting service was developed and extended over a period of several years. The welfare workers visited the mothers at home and advised them on matters of hygiene and housekeeping. In doing so, the (mostly female) home visitors, who of course also had the tendency to moralise, interfered with the privacy of the families.[49] Their paternalism, based on bourgeois values and rules of hygiene, was one reason why mothers considered the infant welfare programme double-sided. On the one hand the welfare workers could give valuable help and instruction, especially to lower-class mothers who often lacked basic knowledge and skills. However, they often proved to be an invasive and critical force within the private sphere of the family.

The Society also offered infant care courses for young women and mothers. Again, their success remains dubious. Although there is only limited information available, the few examples speak for themselves. In Düsseldorf,

---

[46] 'Die neue Polizeiverordnung, betreffend das Haltekinderwesen im Regierungsbezirk Düsseldorf', *Mutter und Kind*, 5 (1913), 7–8.

[47] Vögele, 'Urban Infant Mortality'.

[48] Stadtarchiv Düsseldorf III 4215, 20.

[49] Frevert, 'The Civilizing Tendency'.

the audience amounted, on average, to twelve people per course.[50] Teachers permanently complained about the irregular attendance and a general lack of interest. When asked for the reasons, young mothers stated that they considered infant care to be a natural behaviour, which did not need to be learned. Others felt disturbed by their sense of shame, stating that young girls should not know about these matters ('Und junge Mädchen sollen davon auch schon hören, das paßt sich doch nicht').[51] Similarly, lectures and courses offered in co-operation with local industrial companies or factories suffered from a lack of participants. An official of the Mannesmann Röhrenwerke, a large company where courses in infant and child care were offered, complained that female workers showed little interest in participating. The women stated that they were tired after a long day's work. As they lacked even the basic material requirements to raise the children in decent conditions – so the women continued – they would neither have the time, nor the slightest inclination to attend such courses.[52] It is not surprising therefore, that the audience of the Society's courses mainly consisted of members from other social groups. A teacher's report from Düsseldorf indicated that most participants of her courses came from the 'better working class' (the 'besseren Arbeitsstande'). Domestic servants – rather than factory workers – were the most regular participants.[53] As domestic servants were better acquainted with bourgeois life-styles it might have been easier for them to extend bourgeois norms and values to the areas of hygiene and infant care.[54] Other participants mentioned in the reports were the wives of civil servants, physicians, teachers and priests, and can by no means be seen as members of the targeted social groups.[55] It has to be emphasised, however, that acceptance of these courses improved over the years. An extension of the courses and an increasing participation can be seen after the First World War.

As a whole the success of infant welfare measures was rather limited. The reasons for this are complex. Local practitioners often opposed the centres, as they feared that the free advice offered would reduce their own income. Consequently, they did not inform mothers about what was available at the welfare centres or refer mothers to these institutions.[56] In this sense, the medical

---

[50]   *Bericht über das vierte Geschäftsjahr des Vereins für Säuglingsfürsorge im Regierungsbezirk Düsseldorf 1910/11*, p. 9.

[51]   *Bericht über das sechste Geschäftsjahr des Vereins für Säuglingsfürsorge im Regierungsbezirk Düsseldorf 1912/13*, p. 12.

[52]   Stadtarchiv Düsseldorf III 4276, 70.

[53]   *Bericht über das sechste Geschäftsjahr des Vereins für Säuglingsfürsorge im Regierungsbezirk Düsseldorf 1912/13*, p. 13.

[54]   For a general view see J. Kocka, *Arbeitsverhältnisse und Arbeiterexistenzen. Grundlagen der Klassenbildung im 19. Jahrhundert* (Bonn, 1990), p. 145.

[55]   *Bericht über das vierte Geschäftsjahr des Vereins für Säuglingsfürsorge im Regierungsbezirk Düsseldorf 1910/11*, p. 9.

[56]   Uffenheimer, 'Zwei Jahre', p. 311.

profession blocked an important route to the centres. More importantly, however, – and this has political implications for present-day public health campaigns – was the fact that this approach was based on a significant misjudgement of working-class attitudes and living conditions. For example, medical personnel regularly blamed the mothers for not breastfeeding, suggesting that this was relatively cost-free and therefore mothers actually did not need to go to work. Consequently, health authorities promoted the exclusion of women from the formal economy for the benefit of their children. This was a clear misjudgement of the new demands on female behaviour created by industrialisation and urbanisation. Only the middle class feminists developed a new approach, which tried to combine factory work and raising children. Marie Baum, for example, attempted to establish factory nursing institutions in some of the smaller towns, which were based on textile industries and therefore registered high female participation in the labour force. This initiative failed, however, due to the resistance of the regional authorities. Although many manufacturers were members of the Society, they were not willing to support the female workers. On the eve of the First World War such facilities existed in only twenty-one German cities.[57] In contrast with other countries, care for the breastfeeding mother herself, such as providing her with additional food, remained almost completely unknown in Germany.

Unsurprisingly, the breastfeeding campaigns remained without substantial support and breastfeeding rates continued to decline and reached their lowest point on the eve of the First World War. After the war the Society for Infant Welfare concluded that it would fight high infant mortality by continuously broadening the network of welfare institutions and measures. Accordingly, the Society extended its range of activities to welfare work, and changed its name in 1919 to Verein für Säuglingsfürsorge und Wohlfahrtspflege im Regierungsbezirk Düsseldorf (Society for Infant Welfare and Welfare Work for the Administrative District of Düsseldorf). In the following years, however, a new range of activities was carried out increasingly by municipal welfare offices and less by the Society itself. During the establishment of the controversial Weimar welfare state, the various tasks of the Society were subsumed by the municipalities.[58] As this had been the eventual aim of the Society, the decrease in its duties was no discredit to their work. Instead, the successful implementation of the concepts of welfare, especially for infants, into the 'Weimar style' welfare policy can be attributed to the Society.

---

[57] Rott, *Umfang*, pp. 37–39.
[58] D.K. Peukert, *Die Weimarer Republik. Krisenjahre der klassischen Moderne* (Frankfurt, 1987), p. 132.

Conclusion

In Germany, mortality rates peaked at the beginning of the high industrialisation period of the 1860s and 1870s. Afterwards, urban death rates started to decline until the First World War. The urban disease profile was predominantly marked by gastrointestinal diseases, which also played a major role in the urban mortality decline. As this group of diseases affected infants almost exclusively, an analysis of the levels and trends of infant mortality rates provides further insights. Indeed urban infant mortality rates started to decrease from the 1870s onwards, whereas in rural Prussia as a whole, this did not start until the beginning of the twentieth century. As a result of this, after the turn of the century, urban infant mortality rates were increasingly lower when compared to rural areas and to the national average. The large cities in particular benefited from this reversal. At the same time they were exemplary in bringing about improvements in health and hygiene, including municipal milk supply and infant welfare campaigns. However, the influence of these measures on the decrease of infant mortality was still only moderate. Furthermore, the number of milk depots was insufficient. Sufficient supply and satisfactory quality of milk for large sections of the population, especially for the poorer residents, were not achieved during the first decades of the twentieth century.

Similarly, as the breastfeeding rates continued to decline, the impact of the infant welfare centres was limited. Only the increased breastfeeding rates due to the crises of the First World War had a decisive influence on the decrease of infant mortality. During this period, however, the view prevailed that high infant mortality was unacceptable and must be avoided. The most important causes for high infant mortality were systematically investigated and strategies to fight high infant mortality rates developed. Thus, the foundations of a new approach to infant welfare were established. This new approach drew upon specific welfare societies, which, however, were very often based on bourgeois values and ideas of hygiene and therefore had limited effectiveness in raising working-class levels of health. Attendance at welfare centres was higher in urban than rural areas, but was further differentiated by the social class of attendees, who came not from the targeted working classes, but from other social groups. Although the Society for Infant Welfare, in the administrative district of Düsseldorf, tried to move beyond these ideas, it remained committed to the path established by its early pioneers. Nevertheless, the concept of the Society and its work pointed to a future direction for comprehensive infant welfare programmes. The examples of milk supply and infant welfare centres indicate that the experience of new public health measures introduced to combat the urban penalty with respect to infant mortality remained problematic in operational terms despite the best intentions of the municipal authorities and other interested parties. The fact that during the Weimar Republic the welfare concept of the Society's approach was eventually taken over by the municipal welfare system is perhaps a special credit to its original insights.

Index

Abrams, Philip, 5
Allison, William, 65, 92
anti-tuberculosis campaigns
    Birmingham and Gothenburg, in,
      125–7, 134–42
Arnott, Neil, 65, 92
Augustine, 1

Babylon, 1
baptism, 26
Baum, Dr Marie, 206, 211
Beaver, M.W., 203
Becker, Gary, 170
Bellamy, Christine, 95, 107
Benckert, Dr Henric, 131
Berlin, 181
Biermer, Professor Anton, 115
Biraben, Jean-Noel, 42
Birmingham
    administrative wards, death rates in,
      128, 129
    anti-tuberculosis campaigns, 125–7,
      134–42
    death rates, 126, 127
    mapping, 127–31, 133, 134, 142
    Medical Officer of Health, appointment
      of, 127, 128
    public health campaigns, 10–11, 142
    public health problems, definition of,
      125
    socially segregated areas, 133, 134
birth control
    opponents of, 123
Black Death
    European response to, 32
    measures to contain spread of, 19
    Pope Clement VI, response of, 38
Bleker, Johanna, 109
Böhmert, Victor, 113
Brown, William, 90
bubonic plague *see* plague

Bürkli, Karl, 117

Carver, Dr A., 140
Cavallo, Sandra, 18
Chadwick, Edwin, 7, 12, 60, 65–8, 75, 89,
    92, 107, 146
Chalmers, Thomas, 9
Chauliac, Guy de, 44
Checkland, Sidney, 11
cholera
    early sites of, 96
    epidemic, anticipated, 97, 98
    Liverpool, early reports in, 98
    working-class experience of, 119, 120
    Zurich, in, 114–20
church
    pollution control by, 25–30
city
    histories of, 5
    political arena, as, 5
Conzett, Verena, 119, 120
Copenhagen, 9, 52-58
Cowan, Robert, 65

Daunton, Martin, 13
decline in infant mortality
    breastfeeding, relevance of, 180, 181,
      191, 211
    competing explanations, interpreting,
      174–9
    economic behaviour, relevance of,
      170–74
    economic factors, 171, 172
    explanation of, 167–70
    external environment, relevance of, 168
    fertility, correlation with, 170–73
    German cities, in, 166, 167
    illegitimate infants, 190, 191
    infant care, effect of household choices
      about, 180–83, 193
    literature on, 172

decline in infant mortality (contd)
    mothers, knowledge of, 173, 174
    prediction of, 169
    sanitation, effect of improvement in,
        175–9, 192, 193
    seasonal distribution, 204
    statistical analysis of, 183–92
    summer temperatures, effect of, 192,
        203
    Western and Central Europe, in, 166
Denmark
    absolutist state, as, 51
    Health Commission, 53–5
    plague, responses to, 50–58
    pre-industrial state intervention in, 58
    smallpox vaccination, mandatory, 57
Dennis, Richard, 5
dirt, elimination of, 112, 113
disease
    language of, 111, 112
    social, defining, 124
    urban, profile of, 195–9
    virulence, little change in, 156
Douglas, Mary, 112
Duncan, Dr William Henry, 7–9
    adversaries, 63–5
    career, summary of, 61, 62
    Chadwick, praise from, 65, 66
    cholera epidemic, announcement of,
        98–100
    fever cases, account of, 70
    fever sheds, support for, 74, 76
    health of Liverpool, comments on, 90,
        91
    idol, as, 59–61
    lifetime, reputation in, 60
    lodging house question, 78–86
    Medical Officer of Health for
        Liverpool, appointment as, 62,
        65–70
    mortality rates, approach to, 102–5,
        107
    opposition to, forms of, 63
    part-time appointment of, 65
    public health: battle for, 65;
        contribution to, 87
    public virtues, statement of, 59
    reporting system, 104
    reports by, 62

    salary, 66–8
    sanitary inquiries, descriptions of
        Liverpool dwellings to, 89
    sanitary reforms, approach to, 106
    short- and long-term results of work, 87
    staff, 69
    statistical methods, 87
    value of hospital provision, opinion of,
        77
    work of, 59
Dusseldorf, 16, 200, 201, 205–12
Dwork, D., 203
Dyos, H.J., 5, 95

Ely, mortality rates in, 102
Epidemics
    declaration of as political act, 99
    intelligence of, 96–100
    regulations, 97
    reporting, 99
ethno-hygiene, 27, 36
Eucharist, 26
Evans, Richard, 116

Farr, William, 101, 103
Finer, Samuel, 96
Frank, Johann Peter, 7
France
    plague scripts, 41–9
Frazer, Derek, 11

Germany
    acute digestive diseases, mortality
        rates, 202
    breastfeeding campaigns, 203, 208, 211
    communities in, 195
    infant mortality, rates of, 166, 167 see
        also infant mortality, decline in;
        infant mortality in Germany
    infant mortality, statistical analysis of,
        183–92
    infant welfare in, 205–12
    initiatives, 182
    milk, supply of, 199–201, 203
    Society for Infant Welfare, 205–11
    urban death rates, 195
    urban disease profile, 195–9
    welfare centres, location of, 209
Gezelius, Dr Karl, 131

Glasgow
    public health inspection, 92
Göckenjan, Gerd, 114
Gothenburg
    anti-tuberculosis campaigns, 125–7,
        134–42
    death rates, 126, 127
    health services in, 131, 133
    low-rent dwellings in, 131
    mapping, 131–4, 142
    public health campaigns, 10–11, 142
    urban health problems, definition of,
        125
    urban inequality in, 134
Göthlin, Dr Gösta, 135
Graunt, John, 4
Greenhow, Edward, 102, 103
Grey, George, 96
Guha, S., 176
Gregory, Bishop of Tours, 20–22
Grey, Sir George, 68, 77

Hamlin, Christopher, 6, 60
Hart, Judith, 95
Harvey, David, 11
health
    body's and soul's, connection between,
        24
    community, of, 22
    definition, 21
    dietary prescriptions, 27
    socio-cultural dimensions of, 124
    spiritual, 21, 22
Hennock, Peter, 11, 144
Hill, Dr Alfred, 128
Hocart, Arthur, 17
Holland, Philip, 103, 104
Hunter, John, 60

infant mortality
    decline in see decline in infant
        mortality
    Germany, in see infant mortality in
        Germany
    influences on, 15
infant mortality in Germany
    causes of, 195–7
    decline in see infant mortaility, decline
        in

gastrointestinal diseases, effect of,
        195–7
    married and unmarried mothers,
        differences between, 208, 209
    milk supply, relevance of, 199–201,
        203
    peak of, 212
    regional differences, explanation of,
        198
    seasonal distribution, 202, 204
    spatial differences in, 206
    urban, 197
    welfare initiatives, 205–12
infectious disease
    chronic fear of, 2
    society, impact on, 3
    urban communities, in, 1
infrastructure, expansion of, 145

Jordanova, Ludmilla, 8

Kintner, H., 169, 170, 192
Knodel, J., 173
Koch, Robert, 121, 134, 142

Lambert, Royston, 95
Law, C.M., 4
leprosy
    heresy, of, 25
Letheby, Henry, 81
Liverpool
    buildings, regulation of, 92
    cesspools, 103
    cholera epidemic, 98–100
    epidemic disease, diffusion of, 96
    epidemics, 96–100
    fever hospitals and rural hospitals,
        choice between, 77
    fever sheds, 71–8
    fever sickness rates, 104
    Health of the Town Committee, 64
    health-promoting measures, payment
        for, 64
    immigration into, controls on, 96
    Local Act and national law, conflict of,
        64
    Local Act of 1846, 63, 89–92
    lodging house question, 78–86

Liverpool (contd)
  Medical Officer of Health, appointment
    of, 144
  mortality rates, 100–105
  municipal health authorities and older
    bodies, relations between, 70
  National Association for the Promotion
    of Social Science, papers to, 103
  proper sanitary regulations, need for,
    90
  public health campaigns, place in, 94
  public health machinery in, 63
  public health policy, 6
  public health reports of 1840s, image
    in, 89
  sanitary legislation, inevitability of, 91
  sanitary reports, 94
  social and mortality crisis in, 62
  unhealthiness of, 7, 90
  Workhouse, 73
local authorities
  funds, raising, 152, 153
  investment by, 145, 150
  physical environmental, alteration of,
    160, 161
  public health improvements,
    commitment to, 152
    public health reforms, approaches
      to, 144, 145
  public health share of expenditure, 150
  spending and finance, patterns of, 146
  spending, expansion of, 163
  spending, measuring impact of, 153–6
Local Taxation Returns,
  146, 148, 161, 163
lodging houses
  infected persons and bedding in, 80
  inspection, 84, 85
  Liverpool, in, 78–86
  model, 78, 82–6
  overcrowding, 80
  public health issue, as, 78
  registration, 79–81, 85
  regulation of, 78–80
  unregistered, 80, 81
Luckin, Bill, 12

Marseilles, 42, 48
McKeown, Thomas, 14, 18, 146, 158

medicine
  socio-cultural dimensions of, 124
Metropolitan Board of Works, 152
milk
  Germany, supply in, 199–201, 203
Mitchell, B.R., 147
Mokyr, J., 173
mortality
  ability to spend, effect of, 161
  advances in medical practice, impact
    of, 156, 157
  decline, causes of, 14
  economic changes, contribution of, 162
  economic forces, role of, 156–64
  food intake, effect of alterations in,
    158, 159
  German urban areas, in, 15
  Germany, urban disease profile, 195–9
  housing reform, effect of, 157, 158,
    164
  improved sanitation, impect of, 159
  infant, decline in see decline in infant
    mortality
  life expectancy, influences on, 155
  Liverpool, rates in, 62, 100–105
  physical environmental, alteration of,
    160, 161
  population density, effect of, 158, 159
  public health spending, relation of, 145
  public health, rates as indicators of, 100
  sample towns, rates in, 149, 154
  sanitary investment, impact of, 146
  social and economic variables, 155,
    156
  special circumstances, impact of, 159,
    160
  urban rates, 194
  urban, decline in, 199–204
  Western and Central Europe, decline
    in, 166
Mumford, Lewis, 14

Neill, Hugh, 71, 74
Newcastle, 98
Newlands, James, 60, 86, 92, 106
Newsholme, Arthur, 180
Nightingale, Florence, 60

Paris, 4

Pasteur, Louis, 121
pathogens, bio-cyclical behaviour of, 121,
    122
penance, 26, 27
penitentials, 26–8
pestilence
    moral and natural, 22
    remedies for, 22
Petty, William, 4
plague
    administrative script, 45, 46
    Baltic ports, in, 56
    collective responses to, 22–5
    containment of, 57
    control measures, 31
    control, ritual and symbolism in, 24
    cultural resonance of, 42
    Danish historians, work of, 51
    death from, 42
    Denmark, in 50–58
    early modern France, in, 42
    early modern period, writings in, 41
    Eastern Europe and Middle East,
        outbreaks in, 57
    effective treatments, 43
    epidemics, descriptions of, 43
    Europe, crossing, 50
    France, in, 41–9; meaning, 47
    history of, 41
    language used about, 41, 42
    later Middle Ages, strategies of, 32
    measures to contain spread of, 19
    medical script, 44, 45
    miracles averting, 31, 32
    outbreak of 1711, 52–6
    political script, 45
    prayer, aversion by, 22–5
    prevention and cure, tracts on, 53
    programmes for action, 46
    religious script, 44–6
    scripts for, 43–5
    symbolic freight, carrying, 47
    texts, 43–9
    treatises, 42–9
    Trier, passing by, 19–21
    urban phenomenon, as, 50
    victims, disposal of, 54
    victory over, 47, 48

pollution
    church, countering by, 25–30
    contagious, 28
    death, of, 29
    meaning, 27, 28
    ritual, 28
    umbrella term, as, 27
Pooley, Colin, 144
Porter, Dorothy, 7
public health
    activities classed as, 147
    capital intensive nature of, 147
    capital works programmes, 145–53
    central and local government, interplay
        between, 8
    construction programmes, financing,
        147
    deities etc protecting, 33–8
    diversity in responses to, 144, 145
    economic forces, role of, 156–63
    first national Act, 6
    history of, 38, 39
    infrastructure, investment in, 12
    interdisciplinary studies, 10
    Liverpool, policy in, 6
    local government, avenues open to, 144
        local rescue plans, implementation
        of, 143
    Local Taxation Returns, 148
    market failures, problems relating to,
        12
    materialism, case for, 30–33
    medical pluralism, 32, 33
    miracles of, 25
    monitoring measures for, 100–106
    mortality rates as indicator of, 100
        mortality, housing and population
        rates, table of, 148
    new urban history horoscope, in, 11–13
    object of policy, as, 18
    official and priests, conflict between,
        38
    physical environmental, alteration of,
        160, 161
    political criticism, arousing, 123
        political expediency, as, 9–11
    pollution, countering by church, 25–30
    pre-modern measures, evolution of, 19

public health (contd)
    pre-modern urban responses for, 2
    preventive measures, 102
    problems, objective analysis of, 124
    radical action, recognition of need for,
        143
    religious dimension, effect of, 39
    responsibility for policing, 143
    Rome, measures in, 35, 36
    sacraments, role of, 26
    sanitary programmes, cost of, 12
    social diseases, defining, 124
    spending and finance, patterns of, 146
    spending, measuring impact of, 153–6
    statistical analysis, potential of, 13–16
    strategies for, 2
    Switzerland, reforms in, 109–22
    Talmudic evidence of measures for, 34,
        35
    timing and magnitude of investment, 13
    urban mortality decline, and, 199–204
    urban size, relevance of, 4, 5
    urban, definition, 4, 5
    wealth, relevance to development of
        policy, 12
Public Health Act 1848
    campaigns leading to, 94
    compulsory application of, 90
    condition of Liverpool as justification
        for, 90
    medical officers, need for, 68
Public Works Loan Commissioners, 153

quarantine, 99, 100

railways
    expansion of, 145
Rathbone, Theodore, 81
Razzell, Peter, 147
Renaissance, the, 2
ritual
    pollution, 28
    significance and efficacy of, 18
Robertson, Dr John, 129, 139
Rome, 1
    baths, 36
    pleasure haunts in, 37
    public health measures, 35, 36
Rosen, George, 7, 30

Rumsey, Henry, 104, 105

sacraments
    public health measures, 26
sanitary reform
    central and local government, relations
        between, 93, 95, 106
    diplomatic model, 107, 108
    Duncan, approach of, 106
    government functions, 92, 94
    intelligence, aspects of, 94, 95
    principles and techniques of, 92–6
    progress, monitoring, 107
    urban mortality decline, and, 199–204
Schlossmann, Arthur, 205
Schrämli, Johann Jacob, 115
sewers
    investment in, 150, 151
sickness reporting, 104, 105
Simon, Sir John, 59, 78, 100, 104, 105,
        107, 146
smallpox vaccination, 57
social history
    traditional approach to, 111
social institutions
    origins of, 17
Stockholm, 50
Sutherland, John, 67, 68, 71, 72, 75–7, 99
Switzerland
    disease, language of, 111
    law and order, measures to assure, 113
    public health reform, 109–22
    social reforms, discussion of, 114
    urbanisation, 109, 110
    Zurich see Zurich
Szreter, Simon, 15, 144, 146

Thompson, E.P., 5
Trench, William, 62, 70
tuberculosis
    Birmingham and Gothenburg,
        campaigns in, 125–7, 134–42
    definitions of, 135
    education, role of, 141
    French research on, 135
    fresh air, properties of, 140
    hospitalisation of cases of, 138
    housing conditions, role of, 136, 140,
        141

tuberculosis (contd)
  social and environmental factors, 135,
    136, 139, 140
  social reform measures, 137
  transmission of, 134

urban life
  condition of environment, deterioration
    in, 6
  epidemic infectious disease in, 1
  housing, 6
  negative images of, 4
  public health, 2
  unhealthy reputation of, 1
  urban, definition, 4, 5
urban space
  imaginary mapping, 112
  purifying, 37
urbanisation
  accelerated process of, 109
  epidemics, problems articulated
    through, 6
  living conditions, changing, 194
  organised labour movement, formation
    of, 113
  population growth, as qualitative pross
    of, 195

saturation point, 16
  social problems, redefinition of, 110
  speed of, 6
  Switzerland, in, 109, 110

Vaughan, Robert, 9

water
  cost of, 161
    resource programmes, expenditure
      on, 147
  supply, investment in, 150, 152
wealth
  development of public health policy,
    relevance to, 12
Williamson, Jeffrey, 13, 146
Wohl, A.S., 155
Woods, R.I., 167, 203
Worboys, Michael, 139
Wray, Cecil, 81–6

Zurich
  cholera epidemic, 114–20
  economy, decline in, 118, 119
  political crisis in, 9, 117